Trusted advice

Your **healthy pregnancy**

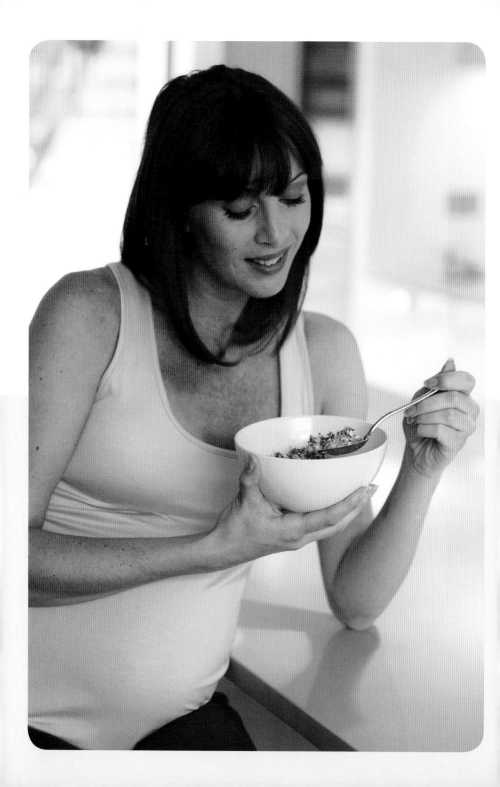

Trusted advice

Your **healthy pregnancy**

A practical guide to enjoying your pregnancy

DRmiriam**stoppard**

LONDON, NEW YORK, MUNICH,
MELBOURNE, AND DELHI

Author's dedication: For Linzi and Will

Revised Edition
Assistant Editor Dharini
Editor Bushra Ahmed
Designer Anchal Kaushal
Senior Designer Tannishtha Chakraborty
Managing Editor Suchismita Banerjee
Design Manager Arunesh Talapatra
DTP Operator Shanker Prasad
DTP Designers Pushpak Tyagi, Bimlesh Tiwary
DTP Manager Sunil Sharma
Picture Researcher Sakshi Saluja
Head of Publishing Operations Aparna Sharma

Project Editor Daniel Mills
Senior Art Editors Edward Kinsey, Isabel de Cordova
Managing Editor Penny Warren
Managing Art Editor Glenda Fisher
Publisher Peggy Vance
Senior Production Editor Jennifer Murray
Creative Technical Support Sonia Charbonnier
Senior Production Controller Man Fai Lau

First published by Dorling Kindersley in 1998
Reprinted 2001, 2006

This revised edition published in Great Britain in 2011
by Dorling Kindersley Limited
80 Strand, London WC2R 0RL
A Penguin Company

Copyright © 1998, 2001, 2006, 2011
Dorling Kindersley Limited
Text copyright © 1998, 2001, 2006, 2011
Dr Miriam Stoppard
The moral right of Miriam Stoppard to be identified
as the author of this book has been asserted.

The advice in this book is not intended as a substitute for
consultation with your healthcare provider. If you have any
health concerns, contact your doctor or midwife for advice.

Material in this publication was previously published by
Dorling Kindersley in *Conception, Pregnancy, and Birth*
by Dr Miriam Stoppard.

A CIP catalogue record for this book is available
from the British Library.

ISBN 978-1-4053-5648-0

Reproduced by Colourscan, Singapore
Printed in China by Leo Paper

Discover more at
www.dk.com

Contents

Chapter 1

Becoming a parent 7

Chapter 2

How to eat when you're pregnant 21

Chapter 3

Exercising in pregnancy 31

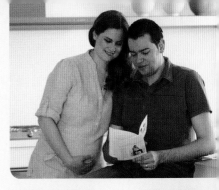

Chapter 4

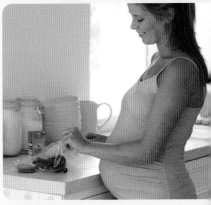

Chapter 5

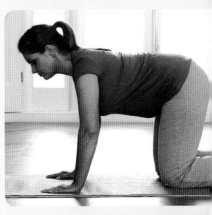

Chapter 6

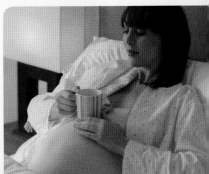

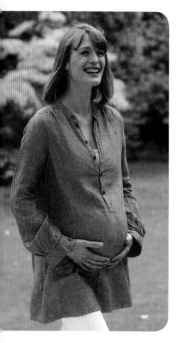

Introduction

When you discover you are pregnant, your excitement will probably be tinged with apprehension. This isn't surprising when you consider the enormous changes that go on in a woman's body to nurture her unborn baby from conception to birth. Pregnancy is not an illness, it's a normal part of human life, but it's sensible to do all you can to maintain your own and your baby's health, and to prepare yourself for labour, birth, and the care of your baby afterwards.

Preparation for birth

Pregnancy and labour place heavy demands on your body, so preparing yourself is important. While there is no special diet for pregnancy, choose a balanced diet with plenty of fruit and vegetables to give you the nutrients you need. There's no need to "eat for two", but eating sensibly and not skimping on meals is important, especially if you are working. It's sensible to exercise regularly as well because not only will you be able to cope better with the extra weight of pregnancy, but you may find labour easier if your muscles are in tone. Learning how to relax and to control the pain of contractions through breathing is also beneficial. The 40 weeks of pregnancy give you time to establish a bond with your unborn baby. Communicate with your baby by stroking your abdomen and responding to fetal movements with talking or singing.

A sensual pregnancy

You may also find your relationship with your partner is enhanced. Due to high levels of hormones, many women find they are capable of greater sexual arousal during pregnancy. Provided that you feel comfortable (your increasing size may make some positions difficult) and your partner is sensitive, you may find this a time of renewed intimacy as you approach your new status as parents.

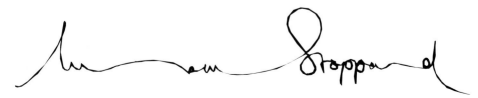

Chapter 1

Becoming a parent

Having a baby is one of the most important events in your life and, ideally, you should plan for it with care. Good preparation will help you negotiate the demands of pregnancy with confidence.

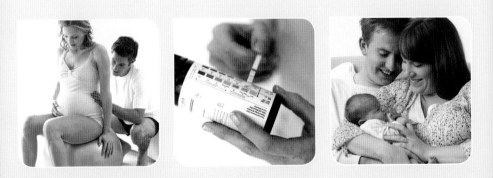

Lifestyle considerations

A successful pregnancy and labour, and the birth of a healthy baby, are the responsibilities of both parents to an equal degree. A baby's health depends to a large extent on the health of her parents at the moment of conception, and her wellbeing can be affected not only by long-standing medical conditions or familial genetic defects, but also by her parents' lifestyle before conception. Many couples do not plan for pregnancy with the same care as they plan for other significant life events, yet it is one of the most important things you can do. Starting a family needs a time of reassessment because becoming a parent will fundamentally change your life.

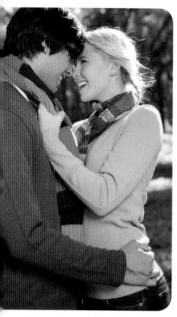

Prepared parents Happy, healthy parents make happy, healthy babies, so make sure you are fit for parenthood before you start trying for a baby.

Changes in your life

All the things you take for granted about your life will be affected by the arrival of your baby. Caring for a newborn is a full-time, exhausting job that will require all your time and energy. However, if you and your partner plan ahead, you will find yourselves better prepared to cope with these changes.

Time Most of us have very busy lives and many new parents think that their new baby will just fit in somehow and life will go on as usual. It won't. Babies and children need a lot of time and attention, and as parents you'll have less time to spend with each other – and with other people – than you did before.

Costs Whatever you earn, you'll probably need to spend about 15–25 per cent of your income on things to do with your child, such as clothing and equipment. But other household costs, such as heating, will rise too, and you may find you want extra items such as a new washing machine or even a larger car.

Relationships It is not only your relationship with your partner that changes when you have a baby. Your relationship with your parents also changes, and you may find that you grow away from your childless friends as you enjoy friendships with other new parents.

Smoking This is one of the most damaging things you can do as far as the health of your unborn baby is concerned, and is the major cause of avoidable health problems. Risks linked to smoking include miscarriage and stillbirth, damage to the placenta, a low birthweight baby that fails to thrive, and an increased chance of fetal abnormalities. A man who continues to smoke while his partner is pregnant risks damaging the health of his unborn baby through passive smoking. It can also have long-term effects – studies have shown that children of heavy smokers are more likely to suffer from impaired growth and learning difficulties throughout their childhood.

Alcohol This is a potential poison that may damage the sperm and ovum before conception, as well as the developing embryo. The main risks to the unborn baby are mental impairment, restricted growth, and damage to the brain and nervous system – well documented as fetal alcohol syndrome. Alcohol can also cause stillbirth.

Research suggests that the effect of alcohol is variable: some heavy drinkers seem to get away with it, while other women who drink only a small amount don't. The only certainty is that there is no effect if alcohol is avoided.

Drugs Over-the-counter medicines should only be taken when necessary, and street drugs should definitely be cut out before you conceive. Marijuana interferes with the normal production of male sperm, and the effects take three to nine months to wear off. Hard drugs such as cocaine, heroin, and morphine can damage the chromosomes, leading to fetal abnormalities and addictions.

Age If you're fit and healthy, your pregnancy should not be any more difficult in your 30s or 40s than in your 20s. However, some problems such as chromosomal defects, for example Down's syndrome (see p. 12), do become more common in older parents.

Hazards Be aware of your environment, both in and out of the home, and avoid anything that could be dangerous. What you eat, where you work, and sometimes who you meet may be risky when you are pregnant (see pp. 56–59).

Diet and exercise Both are vital to your health and the health of your baby. You need to eat a balanced diet with plenty of raw fruit and vegetables (see pp. 22–29), coupled with moderate exercise (see pp. 32–38) because the fitter you are, the better your body will cope with labour.

Stopping contraception

When you decide you want to get pregnant you can stop barrier methods, such as the diaphragm and condom, at once. But if you're on the pill or using an IUCD, more planning is needed.

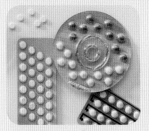

The pill The usual advice is to stop taking the pill a month before trying to conceive, so that you have at least one normal menstrual period before becoming pregnant. But there's evidence to suggest that some women are more fertile immediately after stopping the pill, so this could be the ideal time to try if you've had fertility problems or a miscarriage.

The IUCD or coil The IUCD (intrauterine contraceptive device) works by causing changes in the uterus that prevent fertilized eggs from implanting. A few women do become pregnant while using an IUCD. Even though removing the coil may cause some bleeding, it's still generally recommended in order to lower the risk of miscarriage and infection later in the pregnancy.

Checking urine sugar

If tests show that you have sugar in your urine it's possible that you have diabetes, but it's more likely that some sugar has leaked through your kidneys as their tolerance of sugar is lowered by pregnancy. You'll need more tests to confirm what has happened.

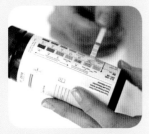

Testing urine Urine tests are simple to do. A chemically impregnated strip is dipped into a sample of your urine. If sugar is present the strip changes colour, and the amount can be compared to a chart that shows glucose levels.

Health considerations

If you have a chronic long-term condition, such as diabetes mellitus, heart disease, or epilepsy, you should not be discouraged from having children. However, you must talk things over with your doctor before becoming pregnant, so that your pregnancy can be managed effectively and, in certain situations, your medication changed.

Asthma This is usually controlled by inhalation of bronchodilator drugs and steroids. There appears to be little risk to the growing fetus from the medication, as long as steroids are inhaled properly.

If you are asthmatic, you need to be extra careful throughout pregnancy because stress and tension, as well as dust, pollen, and pollution, can cause an attack, which may increase the complications of pregnancy. Stress is a trigger, so rest well and try some relaxation exercises.

Epilepsy Research has found that pregnancy has a variable effect on the frequency and intensity of fits, with 50 per cent of epileptic mothers unaffected, 40 per cent slightly improved, and 10 per cent made worse.

Drug treatment must be continued during pregnancy, but you will need to be seen frequently by your doctor, who can adjust your drug dosage. If you take phenytoin, absorption of folic acid can be affected, so folic acid supplements are always given to prevent damage to the fetus. Most pregnant women can change to sodium valproate, which does not have the same effect. If you suffer from epilepsy, discuss this with your doctor well before you plan to conceive.

Diabetes This condition results from the pancreas producing insufficient insulin to cope with glucose (sugar) levels in the body. Pregnancy hormones have an anti-insulin effect, which can worsen diabetes, or cause gestational diabetes. Anyone at risk, such as women with a family history of diabetes, can have a blood test to check. Gestational diabetes can cause the baby to be large, or have heart and respiratory problems, and complications for the mother include chronic thrush and pre-eclampsia. So insulin-dependent women should have their condition under control before conception, and monitor blood-sugar levels closely during pregnancy.

Heart disease Women with a diagnosed condition will be given specialized advice according to its nature. However, as a general rule, it is advisable to avoid over-activity – try to rest each afternoon for at least two hours, and spend 10 hours in bed at night.

The majority of women with heart disease have easy, spontaneous labours. During labour the additional strain on the heart is intermittent and, in total, is less than that imposed upon the heart in the third trimester.

Kidney disease A pregnant woman with kidney disease must be carefully monitored. As long as the kidneys remove waste effectively, pregnancy can continue, but if there is poor fetal growth, early induction of labour will be recommended. (Renal dialysis does pose a risk because the mother's kidneys are unlikely to be able to cope with the additional waste from the fetus.)

Sexually transmitted disease Herpes is only a risk to your baby if you have your first outbreak in the last few weeks of your pregnancy and you have symptoms at the time of your baby's birth. If you have no symptoms, and are not shedding the virus from sores in your cervix or vagina, the risk that your baby will become infected is less than 1 per 1,000.

Chlamydia is the most common bacterial sexually transmitted infection that often causes fertility problems. It may also be transmitted from the mother to the baby during delivery, when the fetus is passing through the birth canal. Testing for chlamydia infection includes a blood antibody test, cervical swabs for culture, and tests on urine. The infection can be treated during pregnancy with antibiotics.

AIDS The outlook for babies of mothers who have tested HIV positive is better than it used to be. The use of oral anti-viral agents should protect the developing baby from infection, and the mother will be scanned regularly to check the baby's growth. Doctors may suggest a Caesarean delivery to protect the baby, and will aim for as little intervention as possible during labour to lessen the risk of the baby's blood becoming contaminated. Although it's not inevitable that the baby of an HIV mother will be HIV positive and develop AIDS, there's a risk that the baby will be born with HIV antibodies; these are usually maternal antibodies and may disappear within 18 months after birth.

Having a rubella test

Before you start the process of trying to conceive, ask your doctor to check you for antibodies to the German measles (rubella) virus.

German measles can cause birth defects, particularly if you catch the disease in the first three months of pregnancy. Problems may include heart disease, deafness, and blindness.

Even if you've been vaccinated in the past you can't assume you're immune to the disease. In some people, the antibodies lose their efficiency after a period of time. If you're not immune you'll need to be vaccinated. After vaccination, you'll need to wait at least three months before trying to conceive, as the vaccine is live.

If you're pregnant and you come into contact with German measles, tell your doctor right away. You will need to have a blood sample taken, which will be sent to a laboratory for antibody testing.

Depending on the result, you might need to have another test 10 days later. If this suggests that you might have German measles, you and your partner will have to decide whether to abort your pregnancy. Some doctors may recommend giving antibodies in the form of gamma globulin to help avoid any damage to the fetus.

Genetic considerations

Down's syndrome

This chromosomal disorder occurs when the fertilized egg has 47 chromosomes instead of the usual 46.

In most cases, the egg itself is defective, being formed with the extra chromosome, or the sperm may be similarly affected. This type of Down's syndrome is known as trisomy. Occasionally, one parent may have a chromosomal abnormality that results in the child inheriting extra chromosomal material. This is known as translocation. Down's syndrome is diagnosed by chorionic villus sampling or amniocentesis.

The risk of having a Down's syndrome baby increases in women over 35 but can also be increased by an older father.

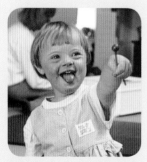

Down's syndrome child One baby in every 1,000 will be born with this disorder. Most cases occur randomly and aren't passed on. However, one cause, translocation, is inherited, so it is important to explore any family history of Down's syndrome.

Within the nucleus of each cell are genes and chromosomes that contain DNA, which determines the growth and functioning of the body (see p. 14). Genetic disorders occur when genes and chromosomes are abnormal. There are three reasons why genetic diseases can occur: a single gene may be defective, there may be a fault in the number or shape of chromosomes, or several genes may be faulty. There may also be complicating environmental factors. A single gene that is defective and results in a genetic disorder can be either dominant or recessive, a mutation, or attached to the X chromosome (see p. 13). Abnormal chromosomes that result in genetic disorders are usually new mutations, although they can sometimes be inherited.

Where more than one gene or environmental factor is involved in producing a disorder, there is as yet no straightforward method of determining why it has happened. If either partner has a history of a genetic disease or condition in their extended family, counselling should be sought (see p. 16). The number of reliable tests for genetic diseases is increasing yearly, although they cannot predict the severity of a condition. If a sign of disease is detected, the ultimate decision about whether to attempt to conceive, to go ahead with an existing pregnancy, or to request a termination will always rest with you, the parents. Bear in mind, however, that although a child with a disability will need special care, many such children are both affectionate and responsive, and can lead happy, fulfilled lives.

Dominant genetic diseases

Fatal diseases caused by dominant genes are rare because affected individuals normally die before they can pass on the genes. However, some conditions, such as familial hypercholesterolaemia (see below), are manageable.

Familial hypercholesterolaemia (FH) This is the most common dominant genetic disease. With FH the blood cholesterol levels are so high that there is a risk of heart attacks and other complications caused by narrowing of the arteries. The condition affects 1 in 500 people. It can be detected at birth by testing a sample of the baby's blood.

Recessive genetic diseases

A defective recessive gene is usually masked by a normal dominant one. However, if both parents carry a defective recessive gene, each of their children has a 1 in 4 chance of inheriting both recessive genes (and therefore one of several disorders) or neither, and a 2 in 4 chance of being a carrier. Thus there are always more people who are carriers rather than sufferers.

Cystic fibrosis (CF) This is the most common recessive gene disorder. One in 20 of the Caucasian population carries the CF gene, and 1 in 2,000 Caucasian babies born is affected by the disease. In non-Caucasians, the incidence is about 1 in 90,000. This disease mainly affects the lungs and the digestive system. The mucus in the lungs becomes thick and sticky and accumulates, causing chest infections. The mucus also blocks the ducts of various organs, particularly the pancreas, thus preventing the normal flow of digestive enzymes. If not treated promptly, CF results in malnutrition. Over 60 per cent of sufferers survive into adulthood, although few are in good health.

Sickle-cell anaemia This is the most common genetic disease among black people (1 in 400). It is so called because the red blood cells are sickle-shaped from defective haemoglobin; this causes the red cells to break down and the small blood vessels to clog, which may result in a stroke. It is usually diagnosed by a blood test. Sufferers are susceptible to meningitis and other serious infections.

Thalassaemia This is an inherited haemoglobin abnormality, which is common among Asian and black people, and people of Mediterranean descent. It produces anaemia and chronic ill health, and blood transfusions may sometimes be necessary. A blood test will reveal the disease and other tests will indicate if the haemoglobin level is reduced. Not all cases are severe.

Tay-Sach's disease Common among Ashkenazic Jews, this is a fatal condition that results in deterioration of the brain caused by deficiency in enzymes. Few children with the disease live beyond three years, and no adequate treatment is known. Tay-Sach's disease is diagnosed by testing blood for enzyme deficiency.

Gender-linked diseases

These are conditions caused by defects on the X chromosome. If a second normal X chromosome is present, as in a healthy female, the defect won't show because it is masked. Women, therefore, carry the disease. If, however, a Y chromosome is present, as in a male, the disease will express itself, as a Y chromosome can't mask a faulty X chromosome. Therefore males are more likely to be affected than females.

Haemophilia This happens when the crucial clotting factor VIII is missing from the blood and results in profuse bleeding from any injury, external or internal. Effective treatment with factor VIII derived from normal blood is now available to haemophiliacs, and they can lead relatively normal lives. Diagnosis can be made from a sample of fetal blood at 18–20 weeks of pregnancy.

Duchenne muscular dystrophy This is the most common type of muscular dystrophy and affects only boys (1 in 5,000) as men with the disease are highly unlikely to live long enough to reproduce. Between the ages of 4 and 10, a boy with Duchenne muscular dystrophy will lose his ability to walk, and is usually confined to a wheelchair during his comparatively short life. The condition can be detected before birth.

Inheriting genes

Half of a baby's genes come from his mother, via the ovum, and half come from his father, via the sperm.

Each ovum and sperm contains a different "mix" of the parents' genes, so each child inherits a unique selection of genetic information, which is different from that inherited by his siblings.

A gene can be dominant (it will always show up), or recessive, with 1 in 4 chances of showing up. So the dominant gene, say for brown eye colour, will prevail over a recessive gene, such as for blue eyes.

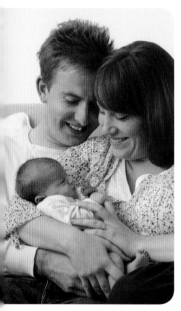

The genetic mix Your baby will have a unique combination of both his parents' genes.

What's a gene?

A gene is a minute unit of DNA (deoxyribonucleic acid) carried on a chromosome, which also consists of DNA. In the nucleus of every cell of the body, there are about 50,000 unique genes divided among 23 pairs of chromosomes.

The "blueprint" of the body

Genes influence and direct the development and functioning of all the organs and body systems. They determine the pattern for growth, survival, reproduction, and possibly ageing and death for each individual. Because all cells derive from a single fertilized egg, the same genetic material is duplicated in every cell in your body (except for the egg and sperm cells).

However, not all the genes contained within a cell are active – it is the site and function of the cell that determines which genes are. For example, different sets of genes are active in bone and blood cells.

Except for identical twins, individuals differ greatly in the composition of their genes, and it is their genes that entirely account for any variation in height, hair and eye colour, body shape, and gender, for example. An individual's genetic inheritance will also determine his or her susceptibility to certain diseases and disorders.

Genes are held in pairs along a chromosome (see below) and each gene is either dominant or recessive. A recognizable effect is the result of the dominant gene or genes in each individual pair; the effect of recessive genes will only be noticeable when there are two recessive genes (see left).

Chromosomes Twenty-three pairs of these thread-like structures are present in the nucleus of every cell, except for the egg and sperm cells. (These cells usually contain only 22 single chromosomes plus an X or Y chromosome.) Each chromosome contains thousands of genes arranged in single file along its length.

Chromosomes are made up of two chains of DNA, which are arranged together to form a ladder-like structure, the sides of which are sugar-phosphate molecules. This spirals around upon itself and is known as a double helix (see p. 15). DNA has four bases – adenine, cytosine, guanine, and thymine – which are arranged in varying combinations, according to the functions of the genes on the different parts of the chromosome. Each combination of bases provides coded instructions that control and regulate all the body's various activities.

Chromosomal disorders are usually due to a fault in the process of chromosome division in the formation of the egg or sperm, or during the initial divisions of the fertilized ovum. Abnormalities of the sex chromosomes result in defects in sexual development, and cause infertility and occasionally mental impairment. Abnormalities can be diagnosed by chromosome analysis, one of the techniques used in genetic counselling (see p. 16).

The double helix The two chains of DNA, which make up each of the 46 chromosomes, are arranged to make a long spiralling ladder.

Chromosome

Each of the four DNA bases – adenine, cytosine, guanine, and thymine – is represented by a different colour

Sugar-phosphate molecules form the sides of the DNA ladder

DNA replication When a new cell is about to be formed, the DNA in each chromosome "unzips" along the centre of the ladder, and each half of the DNA duplicates itself. The new chains created should be genetically identical to the original ones.

Effects of mutant genes

Sometimes when a cell divides and duplicates its genetic material, the copying process is not perfect, and a fault occurs. This leads to a small change, or mutation, in the structure of the genetic material.

Carrying a mutant gene normally has a neutral or harmless effect – most, if not all of us have a mutant gene as part of our genetic make-up. Occasionally, however, it can have a disadvantageous or, more rarely, a beneficial effect.

The effects of a mutant gene depend largely upon whether it is carried within the fused ovum and the sperm, or whether it is a fault in the later copying process of the cells (somatic or body cells).

A mutation in the ovum or sperm will reproduce itself in all of the body's cells, resulting in genetic diseases such as cystic fibrosis. A mutated somatic cell, at worst, will multiply to form a group of abnormal cells in a specific area. These may have only a minor local effect, or they may cause deformity or disease. This type of mutation is usually triggered by outside influences, such as radiation or exposure to carcinogens.

Genetic counselling

Very few couples will need genetic counselling, but if you do, the main aim is to discover how great a risk you run of passing on an inheritable disease to your child. Perhaps you're worried because you or your partner have a blood relative (including a previous child) who has suffered from an inheritable disorder. Depending on what you find out, a genetic counsellor will help you decide whether to go ahead with trying to conceive.

How genetic counselling works

When you are referred for genetic counselling, the counsellor will ask both of you for details of your age, health, and family backgrounds. Virtually every case is unique. The advice depends on a precise diagnosis of a known disease (what it is and why it occurred), and on the creation of a comprehensive family tree that details all blood relationships and any diseases suffered.

Genetic counsellors are also trained in psychology: they will assess the degree of risk involved and help you make an informed decision. If the risk is small, you may decide to go ahead and try for a baby. If, however, the risk is high, you may prefer not to take a chance.

For many genetic disorders, such as sickle-cell anaemia or Tay-Sach's disease (see p. 13), it is possible to establish whether parents are carriers. This can be done by seeing the disease itself, such as sickle-shaped cells on a blood test; by looking for the product of the disease, such as the proteins that are present in Tay-Sach's; or by flagging a gene or chromosome.

Flagging is a sophisticated technique that finds out if a fragment of DNA will attach itself to a chromosome. If it does, the gene, and therefore the disease, is present in your or your partner's genetic blueprint; if not, it is absent. However, in most diseases, more than one gene is involved, so it can be difficult to check all the elements. This is true of cystic fibrosis, for example, although at present the diagnosis can be over 90 per cent certain.

If you already have an affected child, it is important to rule out a cause that is not inherited, such as rubella (see p. 11), exposure to radiation, drugs, or injury. Sometimes it can be difficult to pinpoint the exact cause, but your chances of having another affected child will be outlined.

see p. 13
see p. 11

Can you benefit?

It's important to seek expert advice if you fall into any of the following groups. Not everyone will be referred for genetic counselling, but it's worth checking with your doctor if any of these factors apply to you:

✳ If you've had a child with a genetic disorder such as cystic fibrosis or haemophilia, or a chromosomal disorder such as Down's syndrome.

✳ If you've had a child with a congenital defect, for example, a club foot.

✳ If there's any history of mental disability or abnormal development in your family.

✳ If there's a blood relationship between you and your partner.

✳ If you have a history of repeated miscarriages.

You are pregnant!

Once you suspect that you might be pregnant you'll want to confirm it as soon as possible. There are a number of tests you can have that can be done at different intervals after you have conceived.

Urine tests The pregnancy hormone hCG (human chorionic gonadotrophin) can be detected in your urine. Urine tests can be done at home, and you can easily obtain one from a family planning clinic or a chemist's. These tests are more than 90 per cent reliable. They can be carried out as early as two weeks after conception, although you'll get the most reliable result if you wait a few days longer. Some tests can detect pregnancies as early as eight days after conception, but with greatly reduced accuracy.

Blood test This test has to be carried out by your doctor and is usually only done when there's a problem such as bleeding or pain, or after a cycle of assisted reproduction. The test also accurately detects the hCG in the blood as early as two weeks after conception – about the time your next period is due.

Your antenatal care

You'll have consultations, check-ups, and tests throughout your pregnancy to make sure you and your baby are doing fine. Most pregnancies are perfectly normal, but it's vital to have these checks to make sure all is well and to spot possible problems early.

The antenatal clinic Your antenatal check-ups may be at your doctor's surgery, the local health centre, or the hospital. You'll probably have a "booking in" appointment at around 12 or 13 weeks, and you can expect about six further visits if it's your first pregnancy and about four if it's not. The exact number and timing of antenatal checks varies from area to area.

If you have any complications, such as a multiple birth, a medical condition you had before you became pregnant, or you're at risk for some other reason, you'll have checks more frequently.

Most antenatal care is now handled in the community, so appointments are much less stressful than in the past, when most women had to go to hospital clinics.

Your antenatal records

At your first antenatal visit you will be given a personal file or booklet. On it, details of your personal history (see below), the routine tests, and progress of your pregnancy, as well as any special tests that you may have, will be recorded by your doctor and midwives. This file should be carried with you at all times and you must remember to have it with you when you go into labour.

At the first visit your doctor or midwife will ask you questions on the following subjects:

* Your personal details and circumstances.

* Childhood illnesses or serious illnesses you have had.

* Illnesses that run in your own family, as well as any in your partner's family.

* If there are any members of your family who have twins.

* Your menstrual history – when you started menstruating, how long your average cycle is, how many days you bleed, and the date of your last period.

* What symptoms of pregnancy you have, and the general state of your health.

* Details of any previous births, pregnancies, miscarriages, or problems in conceiving.

* Whether you are taking any prescription medicine or if you suffer from any allergies.

Essential blood tests

At your first antenatal visit, you'll be asked for a blood sample, usually from a vein in your arm. This is used to find out the following:

✱ Your basic blood group (A,B,O), and also your Rhesus (Rh) blood group (positive or negative), in case a blood transfusion becomes necessary. If you are Rh negative, you'll be tested for Rhesus antibodies. Your haemoglobin level will also be checked. The blood test will also show whether or not you've already had German measles.

✱ The blood is further tested for infections in the mother that can affect the baby. A mother who has syphilis can be treated with antibiotics to prevent her baby being born with an infection. The infant of a mother with Hepatitis B can be immunized at birth for protection, and a mother with HIV can be given drugs antenatally to reduce the risk of the baby being infected.

Your antenatal checks

While you're pregnant, you'll have some routine checks to make sure both you and your baby are doing well. Some may be done at every visit, or at different times during your pregnancy. Other tests only need to be carried out once. If the tests show that there is, or may be, a problem, you'll be monitored closely and prompt action will be taken if necessary.

Height Your height will be measured at your first visit. If you are petite, your midwife may suspect that you have a small pelvic inlet and outlet. The chances are, though, that your baby will match your particular physical build.

Weight Women used to be weighed at every visit, but many units now only weigh you at the booking-in appointment. If you lose weight in the first trimester it's usually because of nausea and vomiting due to morning sickness so is nothing to worry about. Maternal weight gain used to be taken as a reliable indicator of the growth of the baby. Recent research, however, shows that external examination, blood and urinary tests, and especially ultrasound scans are much more accurate in measuring fetal growth. A sudden weight gain could mean you have fluid retention, a sign of pre-eclampsia (see p. 70).

Legs and hands At every visit your legs will be checked for varicose veins, and your ankles and hands will be examined for signs of swelling and puffiness (oedema). A little swelling in the final weeks of pregnancy is normal, particularly in the evening, but excessive puffiness may give an early warning of pre-eclampsia (see p. 70).

Urine When you go for your first antenatal visit you'll be asked for a sample of midstream urine to test for any underlying bladder or kidney infection. To collect a midstream sample, you'll be given a sterile pad to clean your vulva and a sterile container. You pass the first few drops of urine into the toilet bowl then collect some midstream urine in the container. You then finish urinating into the toilet.

Other checks You will have your blood pressure taken at every visit, and the midwife will gently feel your abdomen for the top of the uterus to check the size of your growing baby. Your baby's heartbeat will also be monitored at every visit from week 14.

Childbirth classes

I'm an enthusiastic supporter of prepared childbirth and I believe that everyone can benefit from going to childbirth classes. These classes are tremendously enjoyable. You'll make friends and you may find the other members of the group become a substitute for your extended family as you swap stories and experiences, so you don't feel alone and isolated. It's a great help to be able to share what you're going through with people who are in the same position, and it helps to relieve tension and anxiety. Many couples find they make strong lasting friendships with the people they meet at childbirth classes.

Some hospitals and independent organizations offer classes that also incorporate exercise and relaxation techniques – some will prepare you for specific types of both.

Preparation for parenting

These classes are designed to give you information that will make you both feel more confident and are particularly useful for first-time parents. They cover three main areas:

First, the classes go through the processes of pregnancy and birth, including female anatomy and physiology, and the changes that are happening to you and the baby throughout your pregnancy. This will help you have a clearer understanding of what's involved and why things are happening. The teachers will also talk to you about the sort of medical procedures that you can expect, and why these will be done. You'll be given plenty of opportunities to ask questions.

Secondly, you'll be taught relaxation, breathing, and exercise techniques. These will help you to strengthen the muscles used in childbirth, control your own labour, and reduce pain. You will develop the confidence that only comes with being familiar with what's happening. It's bodies, not brains, that give birth, so be open to anything that helps you tune into your body. Your partner will probably be taught how to give you a massage to help relieve your pain (see p. 41).

Thirdly, the teachers will talk you through the stages of labour and birth, and give tips on starting to breastfeed. They'll also give you practical advice on how to bathe and dress a baby, change nappies, and make up formula and bottle feed, which will help you feel more confident about caring for your newborn baby in the early days.

Choosing childbirth classes

Both the quality and approach of childbirth classes can vary – some are tightly structured with little question-and-answer time, others allow time to practise techniques. Some depend mainly on lectures, others on class participation.

You will have to consider antenatal classes fairly early in your pregnancy because in some cases you need to book a place; make plans to start the classes before your eighth month.

The teacher is usually the determining factor, so talk to the teacher and, if you can, check with other couples who have attended a particular class before you make your final choice. Try to select a teacher whose philosophy of birth fits in with the type of birth you'd like to have, otherwise conflicts and confusion can arise later during labour.

Find out how many couples are taught in each class. Half a dozen couples is an ideal size since you will receive plenty of attention from the teacher while getting to know your fellow participants.

In an antenatal class, you may be able to show your partner for the first time, the important role he will play.

By familiarizing him with the processes of labour and delivery, childbirth classes will give your partner the chance to be an effective birth assistant.

Some courses also provide father-only sessions where the men can talk freely about any problems or anxieties they have about the forthcoming event. A nervous partner can find security and support in the company of other fathers-to-be.

Working together Childbirth classes give couples a unique opportunity to work as a team towards a common goal – the birth of their baby – and very often this results in a special closeness between them.

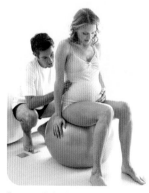

Team work At classes, your partner can learn how to massage your back during the early stages of labour.

Techniques of childbirth classes

Many studies have shown that taking childbirth classes shortens the length of labour. This is probably because knowing how to deal with pain produces a more relaxed delivery. Strategies taught at childbirth classes that deal with labour pain include the following:

Cognitive control This works by isolating your mind from the pain you are experiencing. You visualize a pleasant scenario in which you feel happy about experiencing contractions; for example, when you feel pain you imagine your baby moving further down the birth canal, closer to emerging. In this way, you concentrate on the positive elements of the sensation.

You can also use distraction to cope with the pain, although this works best only in the early stages. To take your mind off the pain, and prevent it from completely filling your consciousness and overwhelming you, try counting to 20, going through a list of possible names for your new baby, or concentrating on a beautiful picture or a piece of music. Focusing your attention on breathing techniques and becoming aware of your breathing pattern is another way of forcing your mind away from the pain.

Systematic relaxation You are taught exercises to relax the various muscles of the body, to decrease your fear of pain and increase your tolerance. This helps you isolate the ache from your uterus rather than allowing it to spread to other parts of your body.

Hawthorne effect This psychological research showed how important it is to have positive attention and motivation. If a mother receives extra, focused attention from a birth assistant, she's likely to cope better with labour.

Hypnobirthing One fairly new approach that you may like to consider is hypnobirthing, where you'll be prepared for birth by a trained hypnotherapist during five or so 30-minute visits throughout your pregnancy. Careful research has shown that hypnosis can help you deal with pain, avoid complications, and may reduce postnatal depression.

Chapter 2

How to eat when you're pregnant

Your body will **never work harder** than
it does during pregnancy and birth. To
maintain your strength and energy levels,
and give your baby the best start in life,
you must **eat well**.

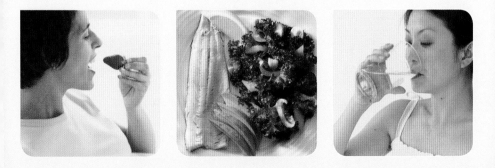

Eating for yourself

During pregnancy and childbirth your body will have to work much harder than it does normally. To cope with the extra demands, maintain your strength, and enjoy your pregnancy, you must eat well.

✳ Increase your intake by 200–300 calories per day.

✳ Start eating 5–6 small meals a day instead of 2–3 big ones.

✳ Make certain you eat extra protein and carbohydrates (see p. 26); protein supplies essential nutrients for your developing baby and carbohydrates meet your energy needs.

✳ Eat foods that are rich in vitamins and minerals, especially iron (see p. 27). These are essential for healthy organs.

Your approach to food in pregnancy

When you're pregnant you certainly don't want to bother about measuring portions and working out how many calories the food you're eating contains. And there's no need to do this as long as you follow some basic guidelines about healthy eating. One golden rule is that the nearer food is to its natural state, the better it is for you. So fresh is best, frozen is next best, and tinned food should be your last choice. It's common sense.

Eating for two?

You'll probably feel hungrier than usual when you're expecting a baby – this is nature's way of making certain you eat enough for both of you. But you certainly don't need to "eat for two" as people used to believe. Most women only need to eat an extra 200–300 calories a day – far less than if you ate twice your normal amount of food.

Much more important than the quantity of what you eat is the quality. Everything you eat should be good for you and your baby. Eating sensibly provides a steady source of nourishment to both of you. Some mothers-to-be, such as those who previously ate an inadequate or unbalanced diet, may be nutritionally at risk and have special dietary needs. More problems develop if you eat too little rather than too much.

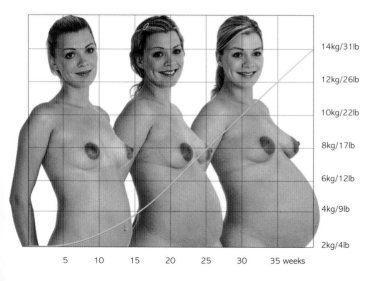

14kg/31lb

12kg/26lb

10kg/22lb

8kg/17lb

6kg/12lb

4kg/9lb

2kg/4lb

5   10   15   20   25   30   35 weeks

Weight gain in an average pregnancy
According to doctors, a woman of average weight ought to gain approximately 10–12kg (20–26lb) in 40 weeks of gestation (see chart, left). This allows about 3–4kg (6–9lb) for the baby and the rest for her support system (placenta, amniotic fluid, increased blood, fat, and breast tissue). There is usually very little weight gain in the first trimester, about 0.5–1kg (1–2lb) each week in months 4–8, and very little in the last month.

Pregnancy is not the time for dieting. Research has shown that when mothers-to-be eat poor diets, there's a higher incidence of miscarriage, neonatal death, and low birthweight babies than normal.

You owe it to yourself, as well as to your growing baby, to eat a diet that's best for both of you. Try to stick to the healthy eating guidelines on pages 28 and 29, but remember that you can balance your food intake over a 24- to 48-hour period rather than at each meal, if you prefer. Just make sure that you don't skip meals.

Your baby's needs

While your baby is growing inside your womb, you are her only source of nourishment. Every calorie, vitamin, or gram of protein she needs must come from you. You're in sole charge of your unborn child's nutrition; you, and only you, can make sure the best quality food reaches her.

You'll be doing your best for your baby if you eat lots of fresh fruit, vegetables, beans, peas, wholemeal cereals, fish, fowl, and low-fat dairy products. A Danish study showed that eating oily fish – such as salmon, mackerel, herrings, and sardines – may help lessen the risk of premature birth. Make your diet as varied as possible, choosing from a wide range of foods.

Don't forget Mum

The other person you must do your best for is yourself. Eating plenty of healthy food throughout your pregnancy will mean that you have better reserves for coping with, and recovering from, the physical strains of pregnancy and the hard work of labour.

Anaemia and pre-eclampsia are much more common in mothers who have a poor diet, and some problems, including morning sickness and leg cramps, may be made worse by what you do or don't eat. Make sure you're getting plenty of natural salts (not added salt) in your diet in the form of fresh vegetables (tomatoes contain lots of natural salts) and fruit (bananas contain lots of potassium).

A healthy diet will help you to reduce excessive mood swings, fatigue, and many other common complaints of pregnancy (see pp. 62–69). And if you cut out or restrict the amount of empty calories you eat, you'll have less excess fat to lose after your baby is born.

Empty calories

The following foods should be reduced during pregnancy as these usually contain nothing more than sugar or sugar substitutes and refined flour.

* Any form of sweetener – including white or brown sugar, golden syrup, treacle, and artificial products such as saccharine and aspartame.

* Sweets and chocolate bars.

* Soft drinks, such as cola and sweetened fruit juices.

* Commercially produced biscuits, cakes, pastries, doughnuts, and pies, as well as jam and marmalade.

* Tinned fruit in syrup.

* Artificial cream.

* Sweetened breakfast cereal.

* Ice cream and sorbets that contain added sugar. (Freeze fruit juice or puréed fruit instead).

* Savouries that contain sugar, such as peanut butter, relishes, pickles, salad dressings, mayonnaise, spaghetti sauces, and a host of other such food products – read the label to check the sugar content.

Your office supplies

It's not always easy to stick to your healthy diet when you're at work. Planning ahead and keeping some supplies in the office will help.

In the office refrigerator:
✳ Mineral water
✳ Unsweetened fruit juice
✳ Plain live-culture yogurt
✳ Dutch or Swiss cheese
✳ Hard-boiled eggs
✳ Fresh fruit
✳ Vegetable snacks – carrot and red pepper sticks, tomatoes
✳ Wholemeal bread
✳ Jar of wheat germ

In your desk drawer:
✳ Wholemeal crackers, crispbreads, or breadsticks, perhaps with seeds
✳ Dried fruit
✳ Nuts or seeds
✳ Decaffeinated instant coffee and decaffeinated tea bags
✳ Powdered skimmed milk for extra calcium in drinks

In your handbag:
✳ Wholemeal crackers, crispbreads, or breadsticks, perhaps with seeds
✳ Dried fruit, nuts, and seeds
✳ Fresh fruit or vegetable snacks
✳ Small bottle of unsweetened juice or milk

What to eat

Quality food is as close to its original state as possible and offers you and your baby good nutritional value. Your goal should be to eat quality food throughout your pregnancy and afterwards as well, especially if you breastfeed.

While shopping, select fresh produce – seasonal fruit and vegetables will be fresher as well as cheaper. Always wash fruit and vegetables thoroughly before use. To avoid the risk of contracting a food-related illness, do not eat liver, unpasteurized cheese, or cook-chill dishes, particularly if they contain seafood or pork (see p. 30). If you can afford it, opt for free-range or organic food products, which are safer because they are free from pesticides and hormones.

Frozen packets of vegetables, such as peas and runner beans, are good standbys – particularly when vegetables are out of season – but canned food should be avoided, except for plum tomatoes and oily fish.

Foods that have been over-refined, such as white flour and white sugar, have had all of the natural goodness stripped out of them and contain only excess calories. Instead, choose wholemeal bread, pastry, and flour, rather than "enriched" refined products, as it is highly unlikely that the enrichment puts back in all that has been taken out. The two "waste" products of refining are bran (the fibre) and wheat germ (the heart of the wheat) and these contain most of the goodness. The addition of bran may help prevent constipation (as long as you don't mind the taste) and wheat germ has a multitude of vitamins and minerals that are beneficial to all. Wheat germ tastes a bit like bean sprouts – crunchy and nutty – and can be added to all kinds of dishes. It is available from healthfood shops, and should be kept in the refrigerator after opening.

As you'll probably have good days with energy, and low days when you won't want to bother, cook up a large batch of meals when you are feeling energetic and store them in the freezer, to be used when you're too tired to cook.

If you are a vegetarian

A number of people do not eat animal products, and many more who are not strict vegetarians limit their intake of meat, particularly red meat. If you fall into one of these categories, you will need to make special efforts to ensure you eat enough protein, vitamins, and iron to meet your own and your baby's needs (see also p. 28–29).

Non-meat eaters can get their protein from eggs, cheese, milk, and fish, but if you do not eat these you will need to make up for this deficiency by eating incomplete but complementary plant protein sources such as pulses and whole grains. These, when eaten in combination, will provide you with most of the necessary amino acids normally found complete in animal forms of protein (see below). For extra calcium, all pregnant women should increase their intake of milk to half a litre (1 pint) a day. (Choose semi-skimmed milk, which has all the calcium but less fat than whole milk.)

All vegetarians need to make sure they take in sufficient iron because there is relatively little in vegetables, and certain substances interfere with its absorption. Eggs and green leafy vegetables will provide some iron, but not as much as you get from red meat (see p. 27).

If you eat no animal products at all, you will have to work harder to make sure that you are not deficient in calcium and in vitamins B_6, B_{12}, and D, all of which are provided by meat and dairy products. Vitamin B_{12} is only found in animal sources; although very little is needed, lack of it will eventually lead to pernicious anaemia, which results in fatigue, dizziness, and shortness of breath. If your diet contains no animal protein, it is essential that you take vitamin B_{12} supplements. Consult your doctor or midwife if you are in any doubt.

Short cuts to a good diet

When you're short of time, energy, or money, eating the right foods can often seem to be too much hassle. Here are some tips that will help you do the best for you and your baby, without too much effort.

✳ Keep a supply of a range of frozen vegetables.

✳ Buy meat and fish in bulk, and freeze in meal-size portions.

✳ Cook ahead and freeze.

✳ Use a microwave oven to cook food quickly and retain nutrients.

✳ Keep it simple – eat raw vegetables and fruit; steam, stir fry, or grill for speed, or bake so you can leave food to cook on its own.

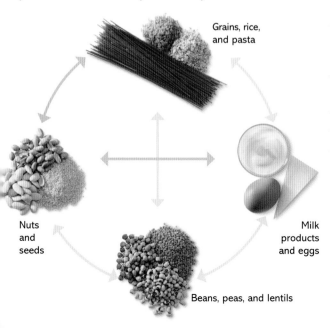

Grains, rice, and pasta

Nuts and seeds

Milk products and eggs

Beans, peas, and lentils

Combining proteins All animal products contribute complete proteins, so called because they contain all the essential amino acids that the body needs in the right proportions. Plant products contribute incomplete proteins, and to get the full complement of necessary amino acids, you have to eat certain foods in combination for example, peas with rice or pasta, or a handful of nuts with rice and beans.

Generally complementary

◁▮▯ Sometimes complementary

Choosing proteins

The needs of your growing baby mean that you'll have to eat 30 per cent more protein than usual right from the beginning of your pregnancy.

This means your protein needs jump from 45–60g (1½–2¼oz) to 75–100g (2⅗–3½oz) daily, depending on how active you are.

Proteins are made up of amino acids, which are vital to individual body cells and tissues. A total of 20 different amino acids are required. The body can synthesize 12 of these, known as the non-essential amino acids, but the remaining 8 essential acids must be supplied by the food you eat. The latter are found only in complete proteins in animal products such as meat, dairy products, fish, poultry, and eggs. Try to buy organic produce, especially poultry, eggs, and beef.

You also need to be guided by what else you are getting from protein-rich food. Meat is the richest source of complete proteins and also contains vital B vitamins. However, some meat, particularly red meat, can be very high in animal fat. Fish can be a good substitute, as it contains complete proteins and is high in vitamins and nutritious fish oils, and low in fat.

One egg contains the same amount of protein as two tablespoons of cottage cheese, one slice of hard cheese, or half a cup of peas or beans.

The important foods for you and your baby

Research has found that what you eat when you are pregnant not only affects your baby at birth, but also appears to have a long-term effect throughout your child's life – even into old age.

Protein

Protein is probably the most essential nutrient for your baby; the amino acids that make up protein are literally the building blocks of the body. Proteins form the main structural elements of the cells and tissues that make up muscles, bones, connective tissues, and also many of your vital organs such as the heart, lungs, and kidneys.

The type and quality of protein in food varies (see column, left). Generally, the more expensive foodstuffs such as meat, fish, and poultry are the best sources, but cheaper products eaten together can also supply you with adequate protein. Whole-wheat bread or pasta with beans, cheese, or eggs; or brown rice or noodles with sesame seeds, nuts, and milk are relatively cheap ingredients that will provide your protein intake. You need at least three servings of protein (see p. 28) daily.

Carbohydrates and calories

Carbohydrates should provide the largest part of your daily calorie intake. As you need to increase your energy intake by 500 calories a day during pregnancy, you should make certain that you eat the best (unrefined) carbohydrates that you can and avoid empty calories.

Simple carbohydrates are sugars in various forms. The most common types and sources are sucrose (cane sugar), glucose (honey), fructose (fruit), and maltose, lactose, and galactose (milk sugars). All of these provide "instant energy" because they are absorbed quickly from the stomach. This is useful when you are in urgent need (glucose sweets may also be helpful in case of nausea).

Complex carbohydrates are the starches contained in grains, potatoes, lentils, beans, and peas. The body has to break them down into simple carbohydrates before it can use them, so they provide a steady supply of energy over a longer period. In addition, complex unrefined carbohydrates (such as wholemeal oats and brown rice) provide fibre, vitamins, and minerals.

Vitamins

These are essential for health. Good sources of many vitamins (and minerals) are vegetables and fruit. Some are rich in vitamin C and others contain vitamins A, B, and E, and folic acid; you must include them all in your daily diet. Many vitamins are fragile, and are quickly destroyed by exposure to light, air, and heat. Some cannot be stored in the body, so good quantities must be eaten every day. Leafy green and yellow or red vegetables and fruit supply vitamins A, E, and B_6 (as well as the minerals iron, zinc, and magnesium).

Although some B vitamins are supplied by vegetables and fruit, the bulk of our vitamin B intake is usually supplied by meat, fish, dairy products, grains, and nuts. Some B vitamins are entirely derived from animal products, so vegetarians must take extra care to make sure they fulfil their nutritional requirements (see p. 24).

Minerals

Minerals and trace elements are essential for the proper functioning of the body. They cannot be made in the body, but a varied diet should supply you with sufficient amounts. Two in particular, iron and calcium, must be consumed at high levels to support your baby's development.

Iron Essential for the production of haemoglobin (the oxygen-carrying part of the red blood cells), iron intake must not only be adequate but continuous during pregnancy. Necessary iron intake varies from woman to woman, and the form in which it is best taken is the source of some debate (see column, right). Bear in mind that iron, particularly iron supplements, can block the absorption of zinc, which is also an essential element for the development of your baby's brain and nervous system. So you should eat zinc-rich foods, such as fish and wheat germ, separately from iron-rich foods.

Calcium Your baby's bones begin to form between weeks four and six, so it's absolutely crucial that your intake of calcium is high prior to pregnancy, and remains high throughout the rest of pregnancy. Foods rich in calcium include all dairy products (choose low-fat ones), powdered milk, green leafy vegetables, soya products, broccoli, and any bony fish such as sardines and whitebait. If you can't drink milk or eat dairy products, you may need supplements.

Getting enough nutrients

During pregnancy, your iron and vitamin D intake should be sufficient to ensure the proper growth of your baby.

Iron The preferred way of ingesting iron is from foods such as eggs and organically reared red meat. These animal sources of iron are more easily absorbed than iron present in fruit and vegetables. It is advisable to avoid liver during pregnancy because liver contains high levels of vitamin A that may be toxic to the fetus.

Foods rich in iron, besides the above, include fish, haricot beans, apricots, raisins, peaches, and prunes.

If you are iron-deficient when you become pregnant, or develop iron deficiency later on, iron tablets or injections will be prescribed by your doctor to prevent anaemia.

Vitamin D This is required to help calcium absorption, so some of your daily intake should come from cheese and eggs – foods in which both are present. Vitamin D can be produced by the body if it is triggered by the action of sunlight on the skin.

* Most pale-skinned people need about 40 minutes of sunlight a day.

* Dark-skinned people who live outside the tropics need progressively more sunlight, depending on their skin tones.

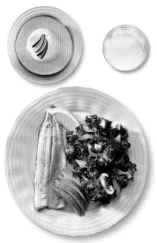

What you need every day

Although there is no need for you to become obsessive about calculating your daily food intake, it is good to have a guide to be sure that you are eating and drinking as well as you possibly can. If you prefer, you can work out your nutritional intake over the course of two days, rather than balancing each meal.

Your fluid intake

During pregnancy, your blood volume and blood fluids will expand by nearly half, so it is very important to keep up your fluid intake. Do not restrict it at all, except for cutting out high-calorie drinks. Water is best, although fruit juices are good, too. If you suffer from mild swelling of the ankles, face, or fingers, do not limit your intake of liquids. It is also essential to keep up your salt intake to avoid problems due to salt depletion.

A balanced meal This meal of trout and salad, melon with yogurt and nectarines, and a glass of milk is tasty and full of goodness.

A healthy diet

FOOD TYPES	SUGGESTED SOURCES	
Calcium foods	• milk or made-up powdered milk • tinned sardines, with bones	• hard cheese • cottage cheese • yogurt
First-class protein foods	• fresh or tinned fish • prawns • beef, lamb, pork, poultry, or offal (not liver), without the fat	• hard cheese • pasteurized milk • yogurt • cooked eggs
Green leafy and yellow/red vegetables and fruit for minerals and vitamins	• plums • mango, orange, or grapefruit • apricots • peaches, apples, or pears	• spinach or broccoli • carrots • peas or beans • sweet peppers • tomatoes
Whole grains and complex carbohydrate foods	• kidney beans, soya beans, or chickpeas • lentils or peas • tortilla or wholemeal pitta • wholemeal biscuits	• cooked barley, brown rice, millet, or bulgar wheat • soya flour or wholemeal • wholemeal or soya bread • wholemeal bread sticks
Vitamin C foods	• blackcurrants • strawberries • lemons or oranges • grapefruit	• sweet peppers • tomatoes • blackberries or raspberries • citrus juice

Vitamin and mineral sources

We are dependent on food sources for all our vitamin and mineral needs, except for vitamin D, which our body generates naturally from exposure to sunlight. The chart below is a guide to the best sources of essential vitamins and minerals. These tend to be fragile, so always try to eat foods that are as fresh as possible.

Sources of vitamins and minerals

NAME	FOOD SOURCE
Vitamin A	Milk, butter, cheese, egg yolks, oily fish, offal (avoid liver), green/yellow fruit and vegetables
Vitamin B_1	Whole grains, nuts, pulses, offal (except liver), pork, brewer's yeast, wheat germ
Vitamin B_2	Brewer's yeast, wheat germ, whole grains, green vegetables, milk, cheese, eggs
Vitamin B_3	Brewer's yeast, whole grains, wheat germ, offal (avoid liver), green vegetables, oily fish, eggs
Vitamin B_5	Kidneys, eggs, whole grains, cheese
Vitamin B_6	Brewer's yeast, whole grains, soya flour, wheat germ, mushrooms, potatoes, avocados
Vitamin B_{12}	Meat, offal (not liver), fish, milk, eggs
Folic acid	Raw leafy vegetables, peas, soya flour, oranges, bananas, walnuts
Vitamin C	Rosehip syrup, sweet peppers, citrus fruit, blackcurrants, tomatoes
Vitamin D	Fortified milk, oily fish, eggs (particularly the yolks), butter
Vitamin E	Wheat germ, egg yolks, seeds, vegetable oils, broccoli
Calcium	Milk, cheese, small fish with bones, walnuts, sunflower seeds, yogurt, broccoli
Iron	Kidneys, fish, egg yolks, red meat, cereals, molasses, apricots, haricot beans
Zinc	Wheatbran, eggs, nuts, onions, shellfish, sunflower seeds, wheat germ, whole grains

Your daily requirements

To give you and your baby the best possible diet, try to include as many of the following foods every day, choosing from the chart of suggested sources (see p. 28). Try to vary the types of food that you eat.

* First-class proteins (meat, poultry, fish, eggs, cheese, and other dairy products) – 3 servings.

* Green leafy and yellow/red vegetables and fruit – 3 servings.

* Other fruit and vegetables – 1 or 2 servings.

* Calcium foods (milk and dairy products, fish with bones) – 4 servings in pregnancy, 5 during breastfeeding.

* Whole grains and complex carbohydrates (wholemeal bread and biscuits, whole grain rice and pasta, beans, and pulses) – 4 or 5 servings.

* Iron-rich food (red meat, egg yolks, apricots, and haricot beans) – 2 servings.

* Fluids – 8 glasses a day, not coffee or alcohol. Water is best.

*Healthy
precautions*

Scrupulous kitchen hygiene is essential because some illnesses are dangerous during pregnancy. Never take risks when handling and storing food, and keep food cold at all times because bacteria can multiply rapidly in warm conditions.

✳ Use clean utensils between jobs or tastings.

✳ Always wash hands after going to the lavatory and before touching food, and take care to cover any infections or cuts.

✳ Ensure that all frozen food, especially poultry and pork, is completely defrosted and thoroughly cooked.

✳ Never let raw meat or eggs come into contact with other foods. Wash your hands after touching these.

✳ Avoid dented and rusty tins.

✳ Throw away any food that looks or smells "off".

✳ Make sure that milk, soft cheese, and other dairy products are pasteurized (see Listeriosis, right).

✳ Do not refreeze food that has already been defrosted.

✳ Reheat food thoroughly only once; throw away leftover food.

✳ Do not eat liver or liver pâtés during pregnancy because they are high in vitamin A, which is known to be harmful when eaten in large quantities.

Foods to avoid

Food safety is important to help prevent illness and infections, so it makes sense to observe certain kitchen hygiene rules and avoid potentially harmful ingredients.

Processed foods Avoid foods containing chemicals – in particular, processed cheese and meats, cheese spreads, and sausages. Do not eat highly salted foods, particularly those containing monosodium glutamate (MSG), which can cause dehydration and headaches.

Preserved foods These often contain nitrate as the active agent, which can interfere with oxygen absorption in the blood. Try to avoid smoked fish, meat, cheese, pickled foods, and sausages.

Drinks Caffeine is a stimulant, so tea, coffee, and chocolate should be avoided in pregnancy. The tannin in tea interferes with iron absorption, so do not drink too much. Alcohol should be avoided altogether.

Food hazards

Certain precautions should be taken because some foods are contaminated with enough bacteria to cause illness, and may even cause miscarriage or birth defects.

Listeriosis Only eat pasteurized dairy products and avoid blue cheese and Camembert, Brie, goat's cheese, or others with a similar rind. These are made with mould and can contain listeria, a rare bacterium. It can also occur in ready-made coleslaw, cooked chilled foods, pâté, and improperly cooked meat. Pasteurizing usually destroys bacteria, but if food is infected and refrigerated, the bacteria may continue to multiply. Wash your hands if in contact with infected animals, such as sheep.

Salmonella Infection with salmonella is often traced to eggs and chicken. Avoid foods that contain raw eggs. Choose free-range eggs and chicken and cook them well.

Toxoplasmosis This is caused by a parasite found in cat and dog faeces, and also in raw meat. It can cause birth defects. Always wash your hands after handling a pet or its litter tray and wear gloves when gardening.

Chapter 3

Exercising in pregnancy

Maintaining your physical and emotional
energy levels during pregnancy is of
prime importance. Exercising will help you
stay in good physical condition both
before and after the birth.

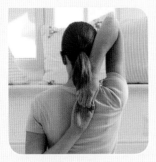
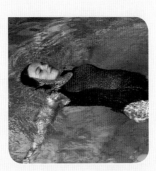
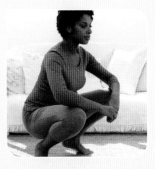

Getting fit for pregnancy

The physical benefits of exercise – improving your stamina, suppleness, and strength – will help you cope with the extra strain placed on your body as it adapts to meet the demands of pregnancy and childbirth. By exercising you can also develop a better understanding of your body's capabilities and learn different ways of relaxing. Exercising increases your blood circulation, and that can also help to ease tension.

Labour may be easier and more comfortable if you have good muscle tone. Many of the exercises taught in antenatal classes, combined with relaxation and breathing techniques, will help you trust your body during labour. Staying in condition during pregnancy also allows you to regain your normal body shape more quickly after your baby's birth. Psychologically, exercising counteracts the tendency to feel clumsy, fat, or ungainly, particularly in the last three months of pregnancy.

How often

Incorporating a daily exercise routine into your busy schedule may not be very appealing. However, many of the exercises recommended during pregnancy, as shown on the following pages, can usually be performed while you carry on with other daily activities. Pelvic-floor exercises may be performed while cleaning your teeth; foot and ankle exercises while sitting at your desk or on the bus; and tailor sitting while reading a book or watching television.

A little exercise several times a day is better than a lot of exercise all at once and then none at all. Normally a woman can restore her energy by resting for half an hour, but it can take a pregnant woman half a day to recover from fatigue. So be kind to yourself and choose an activity that you will find enjoyable and relaxing.

What you can do

You are free to be involved in most sports during pregnancy (until the last trimester), as long as it is a sport you have been doing regularly beforehand, and you pursue it regularly once you are pregnant so that your body stays in condition. There are some activities that are particularly recommended during pregnancy, and some that it is advisable to avoid throughout this period (see p. 33).

Walking This activity is good for your digestion and circulation as well as for your figure. Try to walk tall, with your buttocks tucked under and your shoulders back, and keep your head up. Towards the end of your pregnancy, however, you may find that the pelvic joint ligaments soften so much that you get a backache if you walk more than a short distance. To avoid discomfort, make sure that you always wear well-cushioned flat shoes.

Swimming This tones most muscles and is excellent for improving stamina. Because your weight is supported by the water, it is very difficult to strain muscles and joints, so swimming rarely results in physical injury. Some pools also offer special antenatal work-out classes.

Yoga This has many benefits, such as increasing suppleness and reducing tension. It also teaches you to control your breathing and aids concentration, which is very useful during labour. Remember to tell your instructor that you are pregnant before taking any classes.

Take care

Some sports, such as skiing and horseback riding, should not be attempted once you get big because your balance is thrown out by the extra weight gained during pregnancy, and the chances of falling are high. Other activities, including those listed below, should be avoided because they put unnecessary strain on your body.

Jogging Don't jog while pregnant. It puts strain on your breasts (which need extra support during pregnancy) and is jarring for your back, spine, pelvis, hips, and knees.

Backpacking Weight-bearing activities are harmful as they put severe stress on the ligaments of your back. Also, the ligaments remain stretched, unlike muscles, which can return to their original shape.

Sit-ups The longitudinal muscles of the abdomen are designed to separate in the middle to allow room for the enlarging uterus. Sit-ups encourage these muscles to part even further. The strain may slow down recovery of abdominal tone after delivery. Leg lifts while lying down can have a similar effect.

Is it good for your baby?

During exercise, your blood flow is optimum, so every time you exercise within a prescribed limit, your baby gets a surge of oxygen into her blood. All her tissues, especially her brain, function in top form.

* The hormones that are released during exercise pass across the placenta and reach your baby. Therefore, when you exercise your baby receives a lift from your adrenaline.

* During exercise, your baby also experiences the effect of endorphins, our own natural morphine-like substances, that make us feel extremely good.

* The motion of exercise is extremely soothing and your baby feels comforted from the rocking movements.

Exercise with care

Begin your routine at a gentle pace and gradually build up to a tempo that feels right for you.

Before each exercise, try a few deep breaths. This gets the blood flowing around your body and gives all your muscles a good supply of oxygen.

If you suffer any cramping, pain, or shortness of breath, stop exercising; then make sure you resume at a slower pace.

The joy of stretching

Before beginning any exercise routine always warm up gently (see p. 35) with these few stretching exercises. They will stimulate your blood circulation, giving you and your baby a good supply of oxygen. Repeat each exercise 5 to 10 times. Make sure you are comfortable and that your posture is good.

Head, neck, and waist exercises

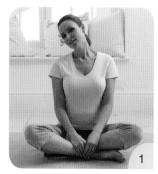
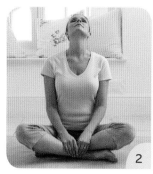
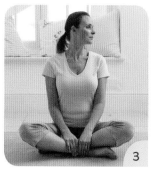

1 Head tilt Keeping your back straight, gently tilt your head over to one side and lift your chin up.

2 Rotation Slowly rotate your head over to the other side and tilt it down. Repeat, starting from the other side.

3 Neck twist Keeping your head straight, turn it slowly to the right, the front, and finally to the left.

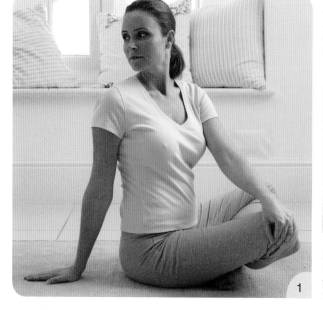

1 Waist stretch Sit with your legs crossed and back straight, and gently stretch your neck upwards. Breathe out and turn your upper body to the right, placing your right hand behind you.

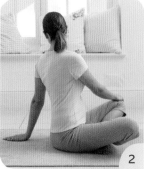

2 Twist Place your right hand on your left knee, and use it as a lever to twist your body, gently stretching your waist muscles. Repeat in the other direction.

Stretching your shoulders and legs

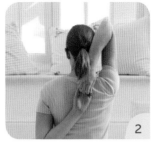

2 Hand clasp Put your left arm down behind your back and twist it upwards slowly. Reach up to grasp the right hand. Stretch for 20 seconds and then relax.

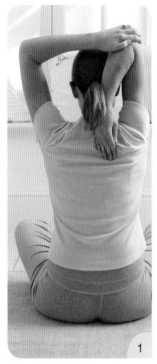

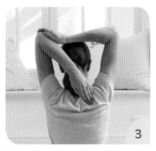

1 Arm stretch Sit with your legs tucked under. Slowly lift your right arm upwards and stretch. Bend it at the elbow and drop it behind your back. Push it further down with the left hand.

3 Shoulder stretch Repeat this exercise with the other arm. Don't worry if you can't clasp your hands together behind your back: just stretch as far as you can.

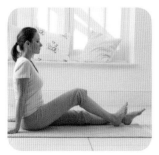

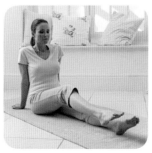

Leg stretch Sit with your back straight and your legs stretched out in front. Place your hands on the floor next to your hips to support your weight. Bend your knee slowly and then straighten. Repeat with the other leg.

Improving your circulation Raise your right foot off the floor and flex it outwards. Then draw large circles in the air with your foot, only moving your ankles. Relax and repeat with the other foot.

A gentle warm up

A warm-up routine prepares your body for demanding exercises. Plan a simple warm-up routine that can easily be made a part of your daily life.

Warming up helps to relieve tension. It loosens up muscles and joints and prevents them from being strained, thus reducing the risk of injury. You may suffer from cramps and stiffness after exercise if you don't warm up.

Choose an exercise routine that you enjoy and that is not too strenuous.

Taking care while exercising

* Exercise on a firm surface.

* Always keep your back straight. Use a wall or some cushions to support your back, if necessary.

* Start your routine slowly and gently.

* If you feel pain, discomfort, dizziness or fatigue, stop at once.

* Always remember to breathe normally – otherwise you reduce blood flow to your baby.

* Never point your toes – always flex your foot to prevent cramp developing.

Your pelvic-floor muscles

The pelvic-floor muscles form a funnel that supports the uterus, bowel, and bladder, and serves to close the entrance to the vagina, rectum, and urethra.

During pregnancy, an increase in progesterone causes the muscles to soften and relax. To counter this there is an exercise you can do to keep your pelvic floor well-toned and firm.

Pull in and tense the muscles around your vagina and anus, as if you are stopping the flow of urine. Hold as long as you can without straining. Relax. Repeat as often as possible each day.

You should begin this exercise again as soon as you can after delivery, to minimize the risk of prolapse. It will tone up the vagina for sexual intercourse, too. If possible, try to make this exercise part of your daily routine.

Exercises for your body

Exercise helps to relieve the strain caused by your extra weight and strengthens important muscles. Learning to move your pelvis more easily during pregnancy also helps you to find the most comfortable position during labour. Janet Balaskas, who firmly believes in active birth, specializes in prenatal exercises based on yoga positions. Some of her exercises are shown here. Exercises lying on your back are best avoided from the sixth month.

Forward bend

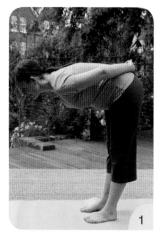

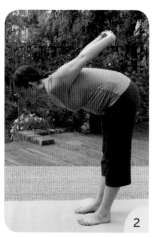

1 Bend Place your feet 30 cm (12 inches) apart. Keep your arms parallel. Then clasp your hands behind your back and slowly bend forward from the hips. Breathe deeply.

2 Raise your arms Keeping your back straight, slowly raise your arms until you're holding them as far above your back as possible. Lower your arms and relax.

Pelvic tuck-in

Stretch like a cat Kneel down on all fours with your knees about 30 cm (12 inches) apart. Clench your buttock muscles and tuck in your pelvis so that your back arches upwards into a hump. Hold this position for a few seconds, and then release, making sure you do not let your back sink downwards. Repeat this manoeuvre several times.

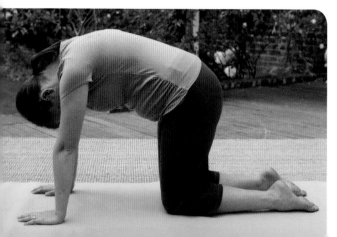

Lower back release

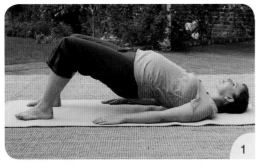

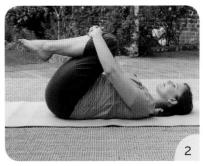

1 Lift your pelvis Lie flat with your arms by your sides, palms facing down. Place your feet firmly on the floor. Lift your pelvis so that your spine rises as high as your neck. Exhaling, come down slowly one vertebra at a time.

2 Hug your knees Keeping your sacrum in contact with the floor, gently hug your knees. Hold for a few minutes, breathing deeply. Do not lift your neck as it may strain the muscles.

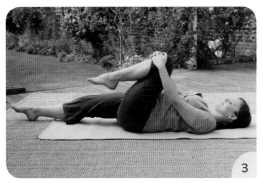

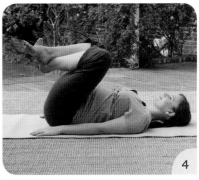

3 Alternate legs Straighten your right leg on the floor and gently lift your left knee. Hug the knee with both hands. Hold this position for a few moments, breathing deeply. Repeat with the other leg. Relax.

4 Rotate your hips Bend both knees and cross your feet at the ankles. Rotate your hips clockwise, making tiny circles with your lower back on the floor. Repeat the motion in the other direction.

Spinal twist

Back stretches Spread arms out flat, perpendicular to the body and with palms facing down. As you breathe out, slowly turn your knees over to the right and your head to the left, gently twisting the spine. Hold for a few seconds. Come back to the centre, rest, and repeat on the opposite side.

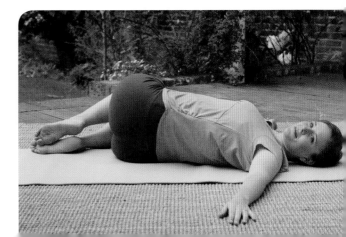

Shaping up for labour

You may have a more comfortable experience in labour if you have prepared your body in advance. Some women find it easier to give birth in a squatting position. Practising tailor sitting will strengthen your thigh muscles, increase circulation to your pelvis, and make the joints more supple. It will also stretch and help relax your perineum. After any bout of exercise, spend 20–30 minutes relaxing. These relaxation techniques are also beneficial in labour, when tension can increase the pain.

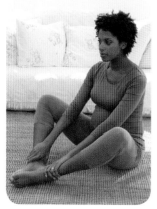

Tailor sitting Sit on the floor and, making sure your back is straight, bend your knees and bring the soles of your feet together. Start with your feet about 30 centimetres (12 inches) away from your body, then gradually pull them towards your body. Open out your thighs and lower your knees towards the floor. Keep your shoulders relaxed.

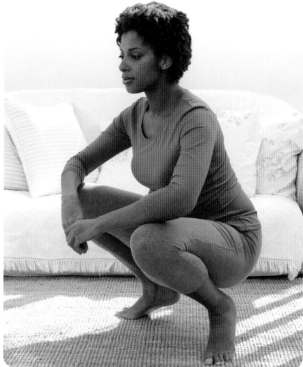

Squatting Stand with your back straight and your feet apart. Squat down as low as you can. Linking hands, spread and hold your knees apart with your elbows. Try to keep your weight even. Hold this position for as long as you can.

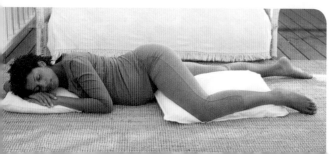

Relaxation As your abdomen gets bigger you may find it more comfortable to lie on your side. Bend your upper arm and leg upwards and place a pillow under this knee; keep your lower leg straight. Lying in this position eases pressure on the major blood vessels and the abdomen.

Chapter 4

Taking care of yourself

The **healthier and happier** you are, the better it is for your baby's development and the more **you will enjoy** your pregnancy. Relaxation, looking good, and feeling on top of things are all important.

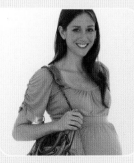
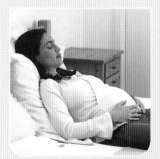
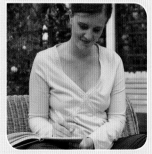

Common massage aids

The lovely smells, textures, and pressures of a massage make it a very sensual experience. Have everything ready before starting to avoid breaking the rhythm.

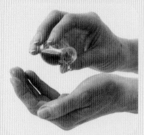

✳ Scented oils help your hands glide over the skin, and leave it soft and smooth. Their fragrance adds to the atmosphere, and makes each occasion special.

✳ You can rub feathers, velvet, silk, and other soft-textured materials on your skin to enjoy a tingling sensation.

✳ Warm, fluffy towels are comforting and ideal for keeping you warm.

✳ Using a soft-bristle hairbrush to brush your hair with light strokes is very soothing and relaxing.

✳ Use a spinal roller for a firm, smooth back stroke.

Gentle massage for relaxation

Being massaged by your partner, or even doing it yourself, is a wonderful way to relax and unwind. A massage stimulates the nerve endings in your skin, improves circulation, and soothes tired muscles, giving you a sense of peace and well-being.

The soothing touch

Use a good-quality massage oil (preferably almond or vegetable oil) to smoothen your hands and skin, and make the massage more pleasurable. Create a comfortable atmosphere by dimming the lights and placing pillows or cushions around and underneath you. In the later months of pregnancy, you may prefer to lie on your side supported by pillows, or sit astride a chair.

You can massage most parts of your body yourself. Massage your abdomen, hips, and thighs with the palms of your hands, using a smooth, circular motion. Work clockwise around each breast, gently kneading from the base towards the nipple.

Massaging your head and neck

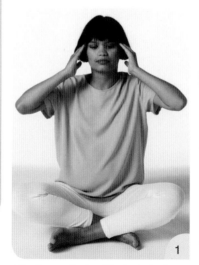

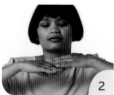

2 Tone your chin Make brisk but gentle slapping movements under your chin with the backs of both hands.

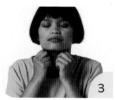

1 Soothe your forehead Put the heels of your hands on your chin. With your fingertips on your forehead, gently draw your hands apart towards your temples.

3 Firm your neck Using your thumb and the knuckles of your index finger, gently pinch the skin around your jawbone.

If you are going to be massaged by your partner or a friend, make sure that the masseur's hands are warm before they start the massage, and that he or she has removed any rings, bracelets, or watches that may scratch or jangle. When you are both in comfortable positions, take a few deep breaths to help you relax. The massage should begin gently and the pressure should gradually increase only if it is comfortable for you. Try some of the following ideas:

Circling Use the palms of both hands simultaneously to make circling strokes in the same direction away from the spine. Lighten the pressure when massaging over the abdomen and breasts.

Effleurage Make light, feathery, circular movements with the fingertips as though tickling the skin. This can be done all over the abdomen during pregnancy.

Gliding Place the palms of both hands on either side of the sacrum in the back, with the fingers towards the head. Push the hands up towards the shoulders without letting the weight of the body fall on the hands. Slowly glide back to the starting point.

Use of essential oils

Aromatic oils can greatly enhance your massage, helping you feel relaxed and refreshed.

These oils are distilled from flowers, trees, and herbs, and are said to have therapeutic qualities. Always blend essential oils with a light carrier oil such as almond. Be careful, though, as there are some oils that shouldn't be used in pregnancy; check with an experienced aromatherapist first.

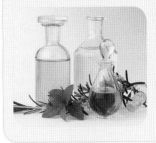

Massage by a partner

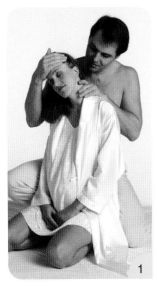

1

1 Support her head Kneel behind her to massage her neck muscles. Gently turn her head, making sure to keep it well supported.

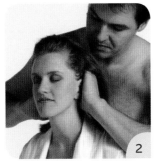

2

2 Relax her neck Slowly stroke the back of her neck with both thumbs in a circular movement. Massage all around the base of the skull.

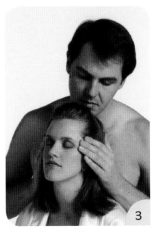

3

3 Stroke her brow Gently massage her forehead and temples. Move your fingers in a light, circular motion from the centre of her forehead outwards.

What do my dreams mean?

Dreams may become more frequent, and even frightening, in the last trimester. There are many common themes reported by pregnant women, and all these dreams express deep feelings and concerns that are entirely natural.

Dreams about losing the baby are usually an expression of fear about miscarrying or having a stillborn baby. Such dreams may be a psychological preparation for a possible unwanted outcome and also a way of bringing your feelings to the surface. In a way, they act as a release for your anxieties.

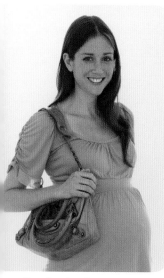

Your changing shape As you get larger, a positive attitude to your appearance is helpful because it will help you to stay cheerful.

How you'll feel

It's not only your body that alters during pregnancy, your emotions will change rapidly too, and you'll experience feelings you've never had before. It'll help if you accept that you will feel upset from time to time – all pregnant women do – and that there are things you can do to help you cope with your mood swings.

Hormonal changes

Enormous changes occur in your body during pregnancy and, because of this, your mood is likely to alter frequently. It is not unusual to find yourself becoming hypercritical and irritable. Your reactions to minor events may be exaggerated, you may feel unsure of yourself and panicky sometimes, and you may even have bouts of depression and crying.

It is normal to feel all of these things because you are less in control of your feelings than usual. Don't feel guilty or ashamed if you show your irritation, anger, or frustration. At work, you may have to struggle to preserve a veneer of calm. This effort will definitely pay off, especially if you plan to return to your job after the birth of your baby.

Changing body shape

Under normal circumstances, it takes some time to adjust to a change in body image, such as losing or gaining a large amount of weight. In pregnancy you are not given much time to adjust to the shape of your body, and you may feel strange about it. You may also worry that you are putting on too much weight and that you will become fat and unattractive during or after pregnancy.

Thinking of pregnant women as fat, and therefore ugly, is essentially an Anglo-Saxon attitude. Many other cultures regard pregnant women as sensuous and beautiful. Instead of viewing your increasing curves with despair, think of them as a re-affirmation of life; see the roundness as ripeness, and glory in the fertility of your body. Feel confident and proud of your pregnant shape.

Conflicting feelings

Even with the most positive attitudes about pregnancy it is normal to have conflicting feelings. One moment you are thrilled at the prospect of a new baby, the next minute you are terrified of your new responsibilities. Becoming a parent is a time of reassessment and change, of expressing and discussing your worries and fears.

The first and most important psychological task you have is to accept the pregnancy. This may sound obvious, but there are women who unwisely go through the early months of pregnancy giving it as little thought as possible, which is especially easy before the baby begins to show.

You and your partner have to come to terms with the pregnancy and begin to think about the reality – especially if, until now, your thoughts about a baby and parenthood have all been in soft focus, a pretty pastel picture of a loving threesome.

Conflicting feelings are sure to surface once you begin to accept the pending realities of responsibility and loss of freedom. Let me reassure you that it's normal to feel this way and you shouldn't worry about it. It means that you are genuinely coming to terms with the situation, and you won't go into shock as some people do when they suddenly have to face all this on the baby's arrival.

Fears

You may be worried about labour – whether you will be able to cope with the pain, whether you will scream or defecate, lose control, or need an episiotomy or an emergency Caesarean. Most women worry about these things, but there's really no need. Labour is usually straightforward and how you behave will be of little or no consequence. You may be surprised at how calm you are or you may not be calm at all, and that's okay too. Just remember that your birth attendants have seen it all before, so there is nothing to feel embarrassed about.

You may also worry about how good a parent you'll be, whether you will hurt or harm your baby, or not care for her properly. These kinds of feelings are quite common and represent legitimate fears. Like many other modern women, you probably do not know much about pregnancy or baby care and may be worried about doing a good job. The answer is to get some hands-on experience – handle and care for a newborn baby if you can. Perhaps you could babysit for a friend's baby, or spend some time with her. If you change her, feed her, and play with her, you will start to gain confidence. Try to get these fears into perspective – you probably had similar worries about starting a new job.

Will my mood affect my baby?

You may worry that your fluctuating emotional changes will somehow adversely affect your unborn baby.

Although your baby reacts to your moods, for example by kicking when you are angry or upset, your changeable emotions appear to have no detrimental effect on her (see p. 47).

On the other hand, your baby enjoys your good moods – your excitement and your happiness. When you feel good, she feels good. When you're relaxed, your baby is also tranquil.

If some activity makes you content and happy, do as much of it as you can and share the feeling with your baby.

Keeping a diary

Keeping a diary at any time of your life can give you insights about yourself that you might not normally take the time to consider.

It is a place where you can express thoughts and feelings that you may not want to share, and where you can focus on yourself. Your child may also enjoy reading it – especially one day in the future when she is pregnant.

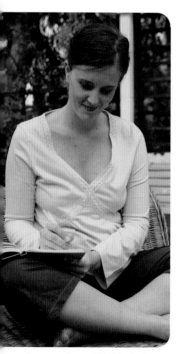

Pregnancy journal Besides having a place to note your progress, keeping a journal helps you to create a cherished record of this special time in your life.

Superstitions

It is possible that you may be more superstitious than normal. Superstition and old wives' tales were, in the past, ways of explaining an inexplicable world. With the excellent medical care now available, your chances of having a child with problems are low, and what you might interpret as a bad omen certainly does not mean that anything will go wrong with your baby.

Coping with emotional changes

Try to see the emotional turmoil you are experiencing as a positive force while you adjust to being pregnant and becoming a mother. Don't imagine that having second thoughts or fears means that you've made a mistake. You're tossing this around in your head the way one wrestles with any big life decision, yet social conditioning makes us feel guilty if we don't walk around with a serene expression. That is absurd. Being pregnant isn't all fun. Accepting the reality is the best thing you can do for yourself and your child.

Spend time daydreaming Imagining and thinking about your baby helps you to form a relationship with her even before she is born, and you shouldn't feel silly if you find that you spend a couple of hours doing nothing but thinking about your baby. Making that connection with the tiny person growing inside you is the first step in accepting your child.

Consider your parents A new baby means a new role not only for you but maybe for your parents, too. Some people see becoming grandparents as meaning that they're getting old, and this can be unsettling for someone who perhaps feels only middle-aged. Try to be understanding and loving with your parents – they might be feeling as confused about their new role as you are about yours. Include them in your pregnancy and share your feelings with them.

While they will, no doubt, revel in their roles as doting grandparents once the baby is born, when you first tell them the glad tidings they may feel they are still too young. Their ambiguous response is natural – their lives are changing too.

Confront your isolation It is quite common for a pregnant woman to feel isolated nowadays. Many women are postponing having children, and some are deciding against it altogether.

You may find that you are the first in your social circle to start a family, and that you don't know any other pregnant women or fully fledged mothers. It can be lonely. If so, look for people to whom you can talk – join parent groups, look up websites for mothers such as www.mumsnet.com, approach other pregnant women in your childbirth classes, and ask your friends or family if they know any pregnant women whom you could get to know. These friendships may provide support long after your baby is born. Don't forget your partner – include him and expand your social circle together.

Communicate Wanting to talk and share what you are feeling and thinking during your pregnancy is natural. Your partner is the logical first choice, and there are bound to be things that he would like to talk about: worries that he may have refrained from discussing with you because he thought that he might upset you, or you might think him silly, or because you were too busy, or too tired. Keep talking. You need each other more now than ever before. Denying or ignoring your fears and feelings won't make them go away. Suppressed feelings have a nasty way of festering and then surfacing when you are least equipped to deal with them, thus becoming full-blown problems.

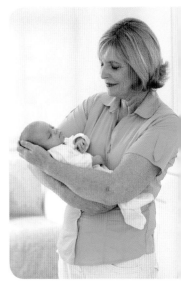

A source of help Even before the baby is born, your parents can often be invaluable sources of information, expertise, and reassurance – they have been through it all themselves.

Coping with material changes

Everyday difficulties that you would normally deal with quite calmly can turn into dramas during pregnancy. Keep a level head, and try not to overreact.

Finances One of the major causes of marital strife, financial problems can become especially troubling during pregnancy. You may find it difficult to cope with an inevitable reduction in income, even if you plan to return to work, but remember that you are in this together. Work out before the birth how you will live on your income once the baby has arrived.

Housing Moving or expanding your home may be something that you are forced to consider – perhaps you need the extra space, or it may be because of the lack of facilities in your area. This can be stressful, and tends to be worse when you are expecting. If you must move – and many couples do, although it's not really recommended from a physical standpoint – do it before your pregnancy is too advanced.

It's never too early to start getting in touch with your baby. What you say, do, think, or feel, even the way you move, may be carried through to the baby in your womb.

Talk and sing Get in the habit of talking out loud to your baby, and singing to her whenever possible. Some children recognize lullabies that were played to them while they were still in the uterus.

Touching Stroking your baby through your abdominal wall is another way of getting in touch and will usually quieten her. In the final months you may be able to distinguish the shape of a foot or hand through your skin.

Thinking Be aware of your baby. Think positive, happy thoughts about her. If you are upset about something, don't shut her out.

Moving Try to move in a relaxed manner whenever you can. The gentle movement of your body as you walk soothes your baby. Rocking and swinging will remain a favourite relaxing activity after she is born.

Emotions When you feel happy and excited, so does your baby. When you feel depressed, she may too – so reassure her that you still love her. Share feelings with her consciously.

Getting in touch with your baby

Being aware of your unborn baby at all times is the first stage in bonding with her and making sure you have a good relationship in the future. Keeping in touch means you'll be aware of what's best for your baby.

What your baby experiences

Even while she's in your womb, your baby feels, hears, sees, tastes, responds, and even learns and remembers. She's not, despite what doctors used to think, an unformed, blank personality. She has firm likes and dislikes. She enjoys soothing voices, simple music with a single melody line (lullabies, flute music), rhythmic movements, and the feeling of your stroking her through your skin. Her dislikes include loud voices, music with an insistent beat (hard rock), strong, flashing lights, rapid, jerky movements, and being cramped when you sit or lie in an awkward position.

Sight Although your baby is shielded by the walls of your uterus and abdomen, light that is sufficiently strong can get through to her – she can detect sunlight if you are sunbathing, for instance. What she sees is probably just a reddish glow, but from about the fourth month, she will respond to it, usually by turning away if it is too bright. The limits of her sight at birth (she will be able to see faces within 20–25 centimetres/ 8–10 inches of her own) may be a consequence of the dimensions of her "home" before birth.

Sound Your baby's sense of hearing develops at about the third month in the womb, and by mid-pregnancy she is able to respond to sounds from the outside world (see above). The amniotic fluid in which she is suspended conducts sound well, although what she hears will be muffled in the same way that sounds are when you are under water. She is also able to distinguish the emotional tone of voices and moves her body in rhythm to your speech, so she will be soothed if you use a soft, reassuring tone.

The sound of your heartbeat is a continual presence in her world and this seems to be something that will have a profound influence on her. One study has found that when newborn babies were played a recording of maternal heart sounds, they gained more weight and slept better than a control group who did not hear the recording.

A mother's influence

The unborn baby first experiences the world through her mother. Your baby experiences not only external stimuli (see p. 46), but also your feelings, because our different emotions trigger the release of certain chemicals into our bloodstream – anger releases adrenaline, fear releases cholamines, and elation releases endorphins. These chemicals pass across the placenta to your baby within seconds of your experiencing that particular emotion.

Babies don't like it when their mothers feel negative emotions, such as anger, anxiety, or fear, for long periods. But short bursts of intense anxiety or anger (caused by a moment of panic or an argument with your partner) don't appear to have any long-term effect on your unborn child. They may even be good for her as they may help her start to learn how to cope with stressful situations in the future.

On the other hand, research suggests that long-term festering anger or anxiety, such as you might feel if you have relationship problems or an unsupportive partner, or if you're living in poor conditions, can be harmful for your baby. The effects may include a problematic birth, a low birthweight, being a colicky baby, and future learning problems. Fortunately, studies also show that if a mother is generally happy and positive about being pregnant and doesn't shut out her unborn baby, any periods of negative emotions seem to have far less effect.

A father's influence

As the expectant father, you are the second most important influence in your unborn baby's life. Your attitude towards your partner, the pregnancy, and your child is crucial. If you are happy and looking forward to meeting your newborn, your partner is much more likely to be happy and to enjoy her pregnancy. This, in turn, means that your baby is much more likely to be a contented, healthy child.

In addition, you should talk directly to your unborn baby as often as possible because research has shown that newborn babies can recognize the voices of their fathers as well as their mothers.

Tips for make-up

Pregnancy can change your skin's tone and colour. You may want to adjust your make-up to counteract the effects.

Fine lines or wrinkles These will become accentuated if your skin becomes drier than usual, so stop using products that make them look obvious, such as shiny or glittering eye shadows, heavy foundations, and coloured powders.

Extra greasy skin To combat this, use an astringent lotion and oil-free foundation, and dust with translucent powder.

Extra dry skin This is rare in pregnancy, but if your skin becomes very dry and flaky, you should avoid using make-up but continue to moisturize your skin. If you must wear make-up, use an oil-based foundation and powder to help slow water loss. Thick, creamy moisturizers act as a barrier to water loss.

High colour and spider veins Stipple a thin, light coat of a neutral matt foundation that is free of any pink on to your cheeks. When dry, cover with your regular foundation and a transparent powder.

Dark circles Lightly dab on a cover-up cream over a thin layer of foundation under your eyes. Leave to dry. Cover with another thin layer of foundation and blend. Dust transparent powder on top.

Your changing body

The pregnancy hormones bring about changes to almost every part of your body, including your skin, hair, teeth, and gums. Moreover, your enlarging abdomen will affect your posture, possibly causing backache and fatigue, so it is important to look after your body and pay particular attention to the way you stand and move (see p. 50).

Skin

Your skin will probably "bloom" during pregnancy because the pregnancy hormones encourage it to retain moisture that plumps it out, making it more supple, less oily, and less prone to spots. The extra blood circulating round your body will also cause your skin to glow. However, the opposite can sometimes happen. Red patches may enlarge, acne may worsen, areas may become dry and scaly, and you may even notice deeper pigmentation across your face, particularly if you have freckles.

Skin care If your skin is drier during pregnancy, avoid using soap because it removes the natural oils from the skin. Try using baby lotion, or glycerine-based soap and body wash instead. Always use oils in the bath to minimize the dehydrating effects of hard water, and do not lie in a bath for long because prolonged contact with water particularly dehydrates the skin. Using make-up is good for your morale, and can also act as a moisturizer for the skin as it prevents water loss (see left).

Skin pigmentation Nearly all pregnant woman are affected by deeper pigmentation, especially in the areas that are pigmented to begin with, for example, freckles, moles, and the areolae of the breasts. Your genitalia and the skin of the inner sides of the thighs, under your eyes, and in your armpits may become darker, too.

A dark line, called the linea nigra, often appears down the centre of your stomach. It marks the division of your abdominal muscles, which separate slightly to accommodate your expanding uterus.

After birth, the linea nigra and the areolae usually remain darker for some time, but all pigmentation will gradually fade and disappear. Sunlight intensifies all areas of skin that are already pigmented, and many women find that they tan more easily during pregnancy. Keep your skin covered up in hot sun, or use a sun block, especially on the face and delicate areas, such as your nipples.

Chloasma This is a type of pigmentation, also called the mask of pregnancy, which appears as brown patches on the bridge of the nose, cheeks, and neck. The only way to cope with chloasma is to camouflage it with a blemish stick or the cover-up cosmetics that are used for birthmarks. Never try to bleach out the pigment; the patches will begin to fade within three months of giving birth. Some black women develop patches of paler skin (vitiligo) on their faces and necks. These also usually disappear after birth and can easily be camouflaged during pregnancy.

Spider veins In pregnancy, all the blood vessels become sensitive – rapidly dilating when you're hot, and constricting quickly when you're cold. Consequently, tiny broken blood vessels called spider veins may appear on your face, particularly on your cheeks. Do not worry – these should disappear altogether within three months.

Pimples If your skin has a tendency to become spotty before periods, you may get pimples now, particularly in the first trimester when the pregnancy hormones stimulating the sebaceous glands in the skin have not yet settled down. Try to keep your skin as clean as possible, and use a cleanser two or three times a day to prevent spots. If a spot appears, do not squeeze it but apply a tiny smear of antiseptic cream.

Stretch marks About 90 per cent of pregnant women get stretch marks. These usually appear across the stomach, although they can also affect the thighs, hips, breasts, and upper arms. Nothing you can apply to the skin (including oil) and nothing you eat will prevent stretch marks because they are due to the breakdown of protein in the skin by the high levels of pregnancy hormones. Gradual weight gain should allow the skin to stretch without thinning, although some women are blessed with more elastic skin than others. While the reddish streaks look prominent during pregnancy, after delivery they become paler until they become faint silvery streaks that are barely noticeable.

Caring for your body

During pregnancy, it is very common to have problems with your hair and teeth.

Your hair The high levels of pregnancy hormones stop the usual cycle of hair growth and loss. Usually, some hair grows and some is lost every day. In pregnancy, however, the cycle is stopped in the growth phase.

After delivery, the growth cycle passes into a resting phase when hair can be shed at an alarming rate. Hair loss can go on for up to two years but rest assured, it will stop – pregnancy never causes baldness. This hair is simply what you would normally have lost throughout the nine months of pregnancy.

Your teeth You're more likely than usual to have gum problems due to the high level of progesterone, which tends to soften all the tissues of your body.

The tiny capillaries around the gum margin often bleed easily. A balanced diet with sufficient calcium and first-class protein, along with a good supply of vitamins B, C, and D, helps prevent teeth and gum problems. Have a dental check at least once during your pregnancy, but be sure to tell your dentist that you are pregnant because it's safest to avoid X-rays.

Avoiding problems

The pregnancy hormones stretch and soften your ligaments, particularly in the lower back, making them more vulnerable to strain. However, with a little care you can avoid the unnecessary problems and fatigue that many women suffer from during pregnancy.

Protect your back

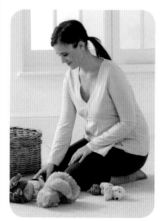

Don't bend down When you are doing household chores or working in the garden, and you need to work on something at floor level, sit or kneel to bring it within easy reach. You can sit back on your heels, but try to avoid making your legs go numb. If possible, avoid bending or stooping.

Lifting and carrying To lift something from the floor, reach down towards it by bending your knees, keeping your back as straight as you can. When you pick it up, hold it close to your body with both hands. When you lift the object, straighten your legs, so that you are able to use the strength of your leg and thigh muscles to do the actual lifting. Never struggle to lift objects that are too heavy – always get someone to help you. Don't try lifting heavy things to or from high shelves. If you are carrying heavy bags, try to divide the weight equally between both hands.

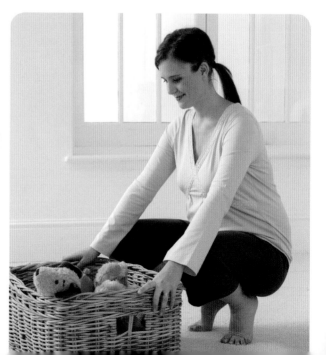

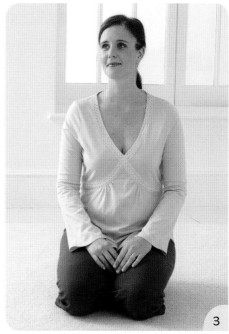

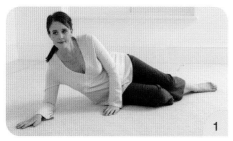

1 **Getting up** When you have been lying down in bed or on the floor – for instance, if you have been exercising – get up in easy stages. First, turn on to your side.

2 **Into the kneeling position** After turning on to your side, use your hands to support yourself as you move into an upright position.

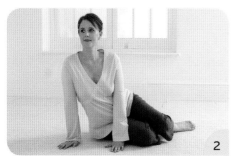

3 **Sitting up** Keeping your back straight, use the strength of your thigh muscles to push yourself into a sitting position. Now you can stand up without straining your abdomen.

Skin and nail problems

POSSIBLE PROBLEMS	WHAT TO DO
Itching or chafed skin The skin of your extended abdomen may become itchy, and the area between your thighs may become a little chafed.	Massage your skin with baby lotion to stimulate the blood supply and ease irritation. Keep the thigh area dry; dust with powder and wear cotton underwear. If the area becomes red and sore, apply zinc cream.
Rashes These are not uncommon in the groin and under the breasts, and are a result of excess weight gain and sweat that accumulates in the skin folds. Poor hygiene will increase the risk.	Keep your groin area and the skin under your breasts clean. Apply calamine or other drying lotion. Take care to keep your weight gain under control. Wear a firm, supporting bra to hold up the breasts.
Pigmentation Many women find that their skin pigmentation alters when they are pregnant; this particularly affects darker areas such as freckles, moles, and the areolae of the breasts.	Use a sun block to protect your skin from the ultraviolet rays in sunlight. The pigmentation effects will disappear after the birth.
Brittle nails Your fingernails will grow faster than usual during pregnancy, but they may also become brittle and split or break more easily than they did before.	Keep your nails short and well trimmed. Wear protective gloves for housework and while working in the garden.

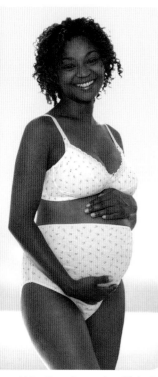

Maternity underwear A well-fitting bra that gives you good support is vital for your comfort during pregnancy – and for your figure afterwards.

What to wear when you're pregnant

Comfort is the main thing where clothes are concerned when you're pregnant. As you get bigger, try to stay one step ahead – there's nothing worse than feeling constricted in clothes that are too small for you. You'll probably feel warmer than usual during pregnancy because your blood is circulating round your body at a faster rate. Your feet and legs may tend to swell, particularly towards the end of the day, so choose your shoes and hosiery with extra care.

Clothes

You don't need to buy lots of expensive maternity clothes. If you have a few specially bought basics – such as a pair of maternity jeans with an expandable front panel, a selection of properly fitted maternity bras, some maternity cotton or wool tights and leggings with expandable gussets, and one or two maternity dresses for special occasions – you can add a few inexpensive items, such as ethnic dresses, drawstring cotton trousers, and comfortable tops and jumpers – some of which can still be worn after your pregnancy. Lots of pregnant women no longer want to wear tent-like clothes, preferring to show off their new shape.

Before you splash out on any special outfits, find out if any of your friends or neighbours have pregnancy clothes that you could borrow. In some areas you'll find shops that specialize in nearly new maternity clothes, which you can buy at bargain prices. It's best to avoid synthetic fabrics if you can – natural fabrics will be far more comfortable. Polyester, for example, tends to trap moisture and is uncomfortable in hot weather.

Work clothes Depending on where you work, you may be able to get away with wearing smarter versions of your casual wear, such as maternity trousers with an elegant top or a loose cotton skirt with a crisp cotton blouse. However, if you work in an environment where formal clothes are worn, you may have to invest in higher-priced maternity suits, or ordinary long-line jackets, large-size skirts and blouses, and drop-waist dresses. If you wear a uniform, make sure to tell your employers as soon as you know that you are pregnant, as they may be able to offer you a larger size if they have sufficient notice.

Shoes

The bigger you get, the more unstable you become, so it's best to wear flat or low-heeled, comfortable, easy-fitting shoes. Make sure they support your feet well, are roomy enough, and preferably have a nonslip sole for safety.

Trainers are ideal – choose a pair with a Velcro fastening because later in your pregnancy you might find it hard to bend down to do up laces. You'll find there are plenty of smart, flat shoes in the shops that are versatile and hard-wearing. Your feet will swell during pregnancy, so choose a size bigger than normal, and avoid anything with a heel. Go barefoot when you can.

Underwear

Maternity bra A good bra is essential when you're pregnant. Your breasts will get bigger, particularly during the first three months, and if you don't support them, they're likely to sag later on. This is because the sling of fibrous tissue to which they are attached never gets its shape back once it's stretched. Go for a well-fitting bra which will help to prevent stretching in the first place.

When you buy a bra, it's best to have it properly fitted. A large department store or a shop specializing in maternity clothes or lingerie will have specially trained staff to help you. Look for a bra that gives you good support with a deep band underneath the cups and wide shoulder straps that don't cut into your skin. Back-fastening bras may be better than front-fastening ones.

Only buy a couple of bras to begin with as your breasts will continue to get bigger, and you'll have to get a larger size later in pregnancy. If your breasts become very big it helps to wear a light bra in bed at night to give them extra support.

Just before your due date, buy two or three front-opening feeding bras so that you can breastfeed your baby easily. You can buy feeding bras at any maternity shop or department store.

Maternity knickers Wearing support pants during the second and third trimester will give you much-needed support – especially if you are expecting more than one baby. By relieving the strain, support pants help prevent backache and support your stomach during pregnancy.

Choosing the right hosiery

Your legs and feet can be tender during pregnancy, due to water retention and your excess weight. Choosing the right hosiery can help with this.

Socks These should be made of cotton or wool and be loose-fitting; synthetic materials don't give and can cut really deeply into swollen feet. In addition, they don't allow your sweat to evaporate, so the skin may become waterlogged and soft. Avoid knee-high socks because these can form a restricting band around the top of your calf, encouraging varicose veins (see p. 68).

Tights Maternity tights (even sheer ones) can give a lot of support and help prevent aching legs. There are many different types available in a variety of colours at maternity shops.

Stockings If you find that you suffer from severe thrush, you may prefer to wear stockings rather than tights. Support stockings, or ones containing a high percentage of lycra, will probably be the most comfortable, although they don't offer the same amount of support as maternity tights. A suspender belt can be more comfortable if it fits on your hips under your belly, but be sure to choose one that is big enough and shorten the straps if necessary.

Tips for your day

There are a few minor changes you can make to your normal working lifestyle that will make your day more comfortable.

Put your feet up Sit down as much as possible, and put your feet up whenever you can. At the office, convert a piece of furniture such as an overturned bin, or an extended drawer, into a foot stool.

Relaxation exercises Practise a few simple neck, shoulder, pelvic, and foot exercises as often as possible when at work. These will release any tension, and help to improve your circulation.

Practise squatting Use the squatting position whenever you have to bend down or if there is no chair available. This will strengthen your thighs, and prepare you to use this position at the birth.

Eat well Keep a supply of nutritious snacks available (see p. 24). Although you may still have feelings of nausea, your urge for food may strike at inconvenient moments. A wholemeal biscuit or cracker and a glass of semi-skimmed milk will be filling, and may help relieve attacks of nausea.

Take it easy Try to take things more slowly. Stop whenever you feel fatigued and try to get some rest every afternoon or early in the evening.

A working pregnancy

Pregnancy brings with it a variety of physical changes and discomforts, but continuing to work can give you the psychological benefit of affirming that pregnancy is a normal state, not an illness. Working also enables you to maintain this important and stable aspect of your life at a time when you may be feeling disorientated by the changes created by your pregnancy.

Your rights at work

Most employers will be keen to help you continue working during and after your pregnancy, provided that you keep them informed (in writing) of when you plan to stop work before your baby is born and when you intend to come back afterwards (see p. 55).

Protect your job Discuss with your employer or your trade union representative your entitlements concerning maternity leave and pay. By law you are allowed time off with pay in order to attend your antenatal check-ups, and this also includes relaxation classes. You may need a letter from your doctor or midwife to confirm the classes are part of your antenatal care.

Protect your health If there is the possibility of your work causing harm to your baby – for example, if X-rays or heavy lifting fall within your area of responsibility – your employer should find you an alternative job while you are pregnant, or suspend you on full pay. To get the full benefit of this protection, you must inform them of your pregnancy in writing.

Adapting your routine

Coping with fatigue while working is an ever-present necessity when you are pregnant. Bouts of morning sickness, particularly in early pregnancy, can make the situation even more difficult. As your pregnancy progresses, the weight you're carrying will cause you to feel that even walking is hard work, so avoid working long hours that leave you feeling exhausted. Over-tiredness will exacerbate any nausea or backache, and you could also find yourself losing concentration. Added to this is the stress of travelling to and from your job which, especially if you use public transport during the busy times, can be very wearing. However, if this is your situation, the solution may be to find out what you can alter during pregnancy. You may, for example, be able to change the times you start and finish work to avoid travelling in the rush hour. If you have to do a lot of standing or walking at work, see whether you can take up a more sedentary role for the time being.

Take it easy Don't push yourself too hard in other areas of your life. Be more relaxed about household tasks – your health and that of your baby are far more important than having an immaculate house. Rest and relaxation are vital during pregnancy and you should allow yourself enough free time for a nap, exercise, and possibly a massage.

Ask for help If your partner doesn't already share the cooking and cleaning, ask him to do so. Maybe you could leave most of the chores until the weekend and do them together. Let your work colleagues know you're pregnant early on so that they are more likely to be understanding of your condition with its mood swings, lack of energy, and the need for a less stressful working day.

Deciding when to stop

Some women happily continue working until they are near their due date. However, many women choose to stop working from their 32nd week onwards. It is around this time that your heart, lungs, and other vital organs have to work harder, and when a great deal of strain is placed on your spine, joints, and muscles. You should get rest whenever possible, and that is often difficult if you continue working.

Deciding when to return

Once you have your baby, you may wish to go back to work under different conditions, and you will have to discuss this with your employer – preferably before you are due to return. If there is a provision for part-time employment, or a phased return that allows you to be, in effect, a part-time worker for some time after your baby's birth, these are ideal solutions. You could also investigate job sharing, flexible hours, or working from home in a freelance capacity. If these options are not available, you will need to consider what full-time childcare you can find in your area (and the costs) before you decide on returning to work.

Your baby's safety

Try to be aware of any hazards in your workplace that may potentially harm your baby (see p. 58). If you are worried, talk to your doctor and your employer about the risks, and take steps to avoid them.

A few pregnant women working in offices are still worried about the possible dangers of exposure to radiation from copying machines and computers. However, research shows that these low levels of radiation won't harm your baby.

No workplace should allow smoking indoors. Avoid places where people smoke because passive smoking (inhaling cigarette smoke in the atmosphere) is just as bad for you and your baby as smoking cigarettes yourself.

Drugs and your baby

Consult your doctor before taking any drug, and always let him know that you're pregnant.

Avoid taking any medication during pregnancy unless your doctor determines that its benefits outweigh the risk to the fetus. The long-term effects of many drugs on the unborn child are largely unknown. Some drugs have been proven to affect the fetus, and should be completely avoided (see below).

Avoiding hazards

Many of our normal activities may pose dangers during pregnancy. Cleaning out cat litter at home, or contact with harmful chemicals at work, passive smoking while socializing, or having vaccinations for travelling may affect the development of the unborn baby, so certain precautions should be taken.

At home

Very few of us can move to a perfect environment while pregnant, but you should try to avoid handling raw meat, touching other people's pets and cleaning out litter trays, breathing in exhaust gases from cars, and working with pesticides in the garden. Alcohol, coffee, and teas containing caffeine are also best avoided. Most herbal teas are generally safe (although you should always check this; avoid raspberry leaf, which is said to trigger contractions). Choose organic ones to avoid the risk of pesticides.

How drugs can affect your baby

DRUG	USE	IS IT SAFE FOR MY BABY?
Amphetamines	Stimulants	May cause heart defects and blood diseases
Anabolic steroids	Body building	Can have a masculinizing effect on a female fetus
Tetracycline	Treats acne	Can colour first and permanent teeth yellow
Streptomycin	Treats tuberculosis	Can cause deafness in infants
Antihistamines	Allergies/travel sickness	Some cause malformations
Anti-nausea drugs	Combat nausea	May cause malformations
Diuretics	Rid body of excess fluid	Can cause fetal blood disorders
Narcotics (such as morphine)	Painkillers	Addictive; baby may suffer withdrawal symptoms
Paracetamol	Reduces pain and fever	Safe in small doses
LSD, cannabis	Recreational	Risk of chromosomal damage and miscarriage
Anti-inflammatories (such as ibuprofen)	Relieve pain and inflammation	Can cause premature closing of valve in your baby's circulation system
Aspirin	Pain relief	Best avoided in large, painkilling doses, although it may be prescribed for specific conditions
Antibiotics	Fighting infections	Can be taken, barring some specific types; remind your doctor you are pregnant during consultation

Harmful chemicals You should limit your use of aerosol sprays in the home: there are less harmful alternatives to most aerosols on the market today. Although few modern aerosols contain substances that have been implicated in causing harm to the fetus or the mother, my feeling is that we are all exposed to invisible sources of potentially harmful chemicals, and it's wise to take every possible precaution.

Avoid substances that give off vapour, such as solvent-based glue and petrol, as the fumes they give off may be toxic and should never be inhaled, whether you are pregnant or not. Read the label of any material you use, and avoid those that are potentially harmful.

Some examples are cleaning fluids, contact cement, creosote, volatile paint, lacquers, thinners, some glues, and oven cleaner. Colouring or perming your hair is probably safe, but if you have fears about the long-term effects of the chemicals involved, I would advise you to wait until after the first three months, when the most crucial organs in your baby's body will have formed.

Hot baths Saunas and hot tubs have been implicated in fetal abnormalities, particularly those of the baby's nervous system, in exactly the same way as fever. When your body is subjected to extreme heat over a lengthy period, you can become overheated and this may affect your baby. Avoid saunas and hot tubs, especially in the first trimester, and keep bath temperatures moderate.

Television rays These have not been shown to form ionizing radiation. It won't do you any harm to sit within several feet of the screen, even for long periods. However, make sure you are sitting comfortably to avoid getting backache.

Immunizations Because your entire immune system is changing under the influence of your pregnancy and may be weakened, your responses to various immunizations can be unpredictable.

Your doctor will discuss with you any immunizations that are necessary if you have been exposed to infectious diseases or if you have to travel outside the country. In general, vaccinations that are prepared using live viruses – including those for measles, rubella (German measles), mumps, and yellow fever – are best avoided.

Toxoplasmosis and your baby

This disease, caused by the organism toxoplasma, produces only mild flu-like symptoms in adults, but can seriously damage the unborn child.

During pregnancy the disease can cause fetal brain damage and blindness and may even be fatal. The greatest danger is during the third trimester.

Toxoplasma is carried in the faeces of infected animals, especially cats, but most people contract it by eating under-cooked meat. About 80 per cent of the population have had it and have developed antibodies, but the younger you are, the less likely you are to be immune. You can go for a blood test to be sure.

Guidelines to follow:

✳ Don't eat raw or under-cooked meat, especially pork, poultry, or steak. Cook meat to an internal temperature of at least 55°C/131°F, at which the bacteria are killed.

✳ Don't feed raw meat to your pets. Keep their food bowls apart. Wash your hands after feeding.

✳ Don't garden in soil that has been used by cats for litter. Wear gloves while gardening.

✳ Don't stroke or kiss other people's pets (particularly cats).

✳ If emptying your pet's litter trays is unavoidable, make sure that you wear gloves and wash your hands with a mild disinfectant afterwards.

Your risk of infection

In the first 12 weeks of pregnancy, try to avoid contact with anyone, especially a child, who has a high fever, even if the fever is not thought to be caused by rubella (see p.11).

If you contract mumps during pregnancy, it will run the same course as when not pregnant. There is a minimal but increased risk of miscarriage if you get it in the first 12 weeks of pregnancy. The mumps vaccine is not given during pregnancy as it is "live" and could affect the fetus.

Chickenpox is an uncommon disease in adults. But if you have been in contact with someone who has chickenpox, contact your midwife or doctor. In most cases, you will already be immune, but if not, you can be given treatment to prevent the baby from being affected.

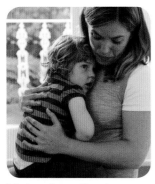

Infectious diseases If you have children, you can't do much to keep away from them. If you are a teacher, send home any feverish child.

Hazards at work

If you work outside the home, you may have many questions that have no simple answers: How safe is my workplace? Will the demands of my job put my pregnancy at risk? How long can I work?

If your job is particularly strenuous, involving a lot of standing, walking, lifting, or climbing, it may be hard for you to have enough rest, making you feel tired during your pregnancy.

In all circumstances, pregnant women must avoid any activity that exposes them to physical danger, including active police work, motorcycle racing, and so on.

Your doctor may also suggest that it's safest for you to stop working if you have certain diseases, such as a heart condition, have a history of more than one premature baby or miscarriage, or if you're expecting more than one baby. Women who are suffering from pre-eclampsia or placenta praevia may also be advised to stop work.

At work, watch out for anything that could be potentially harmful and make sure your employer transfers you to a hazard-free working place or job. Especially avoid:

✳ Chemicals used in manufacturing and other industries – for example, lead, mercury, vinyl chloride, dry cleaning fluids, paint fumes, and solvents.

✳ Animals, which present a risk of toxoplasmosis (see p. 57).

✳ Exposure to infectious diseases, especially those involving childhood rashes.

✳ Exposure to toxic wastes of any kind.

✳ Exposure to cigarette smoke (passive smoking), which can happen in public places that do not have smoking restrictions.

✳ Unacceptable levels of ionizing radiation (these are now strictly monitored by government regulation). It's generally accepted that day-to-day exposure to ultraviolet or infra-red radiation given off by equipment such as printers, photocopiers, and computer screens is not dangerous to you or your baby. But just to be extra careful if you make photocopies every day, it's a good idea to keep the top of the photocopier closed while the machine is copying.

Otherwise, if you're a healthy woman with a normal pregnancy and working in a job with no hazards greater than those you meet in everyday life, you can usually work until close to your expected delivery date.

Socializing

Infections are caught from people with whom we come into contact. Although being pregnant doesn't mean that you should become a hermit, or wear a gauze mask when talking to people, it pays to be cautious – especially around children (see p. 58), or adults who are running a raised temperature.

Normal colds and flu will not harm your baby, but do your best to avoid running a fever. If your temperature does go very high, using a damp sponge and a fan might help to cool the skin sufficiently. Otherwise, ask your doctor's advice on what medications are safe for fever, colds, and flu.

Travelling

There is absolutely no evidence that travel speeds up labour or leads to miscarriage or any other complication of pregnancy. You should only be extra cautious if you have miscarried before, or have a history of premature labour. For long stays, you should ask your doctor for the name of an obstetrician you can consult in the area you are visiting, in case of an emergency. In the last trimester, limit yourself to trips within 30 miles (48 kilometres) of home.

Trains Book a seat if possible, and make sure that it is not next to the buffet car as the smell of food may make you feel nauseous. Eat lightly to minimize motion sickness.

Cars Get out of the car at regular intervals and have a short walk to aid circulation. Always fasten your seat belt, but buckle it low, across your pelvis, and use a shoulder harness if you have one. You can do the driving as long as you are comfortable behind the wheel, but you must stop if you begin to feel cramped. Obviously, don't drive yourself to the hospital if you are in labour!

Air travel After your seventh month, air travel is not a good idea because of pressure changes in the cabin. If you must fly, check with the airline about whether they require a doctor's letter to let you on the plane after your seventh month. Do not fly in small private planes that do not have pressurized cabins.

If you sit over the wings or towards the front of a plane you will feel less of the plane's motion, which can help if you suffer from motion sickness.

Travelling in comfort

While travelling, bear in mind a few important points that can ensure a more relaxed experience.

* Leave more than enough time for your journey, allowing yourself a comfortable margin between any connections you might have to make.

* Travel in short bursts rather than for long stretches.

* Carry a drink, such as fruit juice or milk, in a flask.

* Take nutritious portable food, such as wholemeal crackers, fruit or vegetables, and nibbles including dried fruit, nuts, and seeds.

* If nausea is a problem, carry glucose sweets to help prevent low blood sugar.

Foreign travel
* Take care while eating out. Follow the guidelines to avoid listeriosis and other food-related diseases (see p. 30). Drink bottled water if in doubt.

* Check with your doctor which immunizations are safe (typhoid vaccinations, for example, could harm the baby but the cholera vaccine may not be harmful and you may need it to satisfy requirements in Southeast Asia).

* Rabies and tetanus vaccinations may be necessary, particularly if there is any indication of exposure.

Sleeping soundly

A good night's sleep is one of your top priorities in the late stages of pregnancy.

Aim to get eight hours of sleep a night. However, you may suffer from irritating insomnia because, although your metabolism slows down at night, your baby's does not. It keeps hammering away all through the night hours. If you cannot sleep, there are a number of remedies you can try:

✳ A warm bath before going to bed is very relaxing and makes you sleepy and tranquil.

✳ A hot milky drink at bedtime will help you drop off. You can also induce sleep by reading a calming book or listening to soothing music.

✳ Deep breathing exercises and relaxation techniques are excellent treatments for insomnia.

✳ Instead of worrying about your lack of sleep, get up and do something – maybe a job that has been put off for some time.

✳ If you have worries that are stopping you from sleeping, to help clear your mind visualize each one written on a piece of paper, then mentally crumple the paper up and throw it away.

Getting enough rest and relaxation

With the progress of your pregnancy, you may find it increasingly hard to get comfortable. As your abdomen gets larger, sitting or lying in your usual positions becomes uncomfortable. If you lie flat on your back, the weight of your growing baby presses down on the major blood vessels and nerves that lie against the spine, possibly causing numbness and tingling pain, and even dizziness and shortness of breath. Lying on your side may be an answer, or use pillows for support.

Tense-and-relax technique

A good way to relax your body is to use the tense-and-relax technique. This is a pleasant aid to relaxation during pregnancy, and useful preparation for labour, when it is a great help to be able to relax most of the muscles in your body so that your uterus contracts without the rest of your body tensing.

Find a comfortable position lying on your back propped up with cushions (see below). Close your eyes. Try to clear your mind of any anxieties by breathing in and out slowly and regularly and concentrating all your attention on your breathing. When your mind is relaxed and your breathing deep and regular, begin the tense-and-relax routine. Work through one side of your upper body, then the other, tensing and relaxing each muscle. Roll your knees outwards, then tense and relax your buttocks, thighs, calves, and feet. Finally, tense then relax the muscles of your face, eyes, and forehead.

Your partner can help by touching you where he can see you are tensing up: you respond to his touch by relaxing. It is best to practise this twice a day for 15–20 minutes if you can.

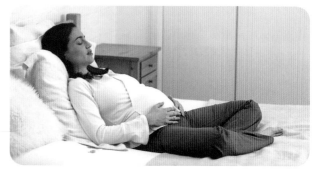

Resting on your back If you can't rest lying on your side prop yourself up with plenty of pillows.

Chapter 5

Health problems

Very few women go through pregnancy without suffering some complaint or ailment. These **can be worrying,** but they are, in the main, uncomfortable rather than serious.

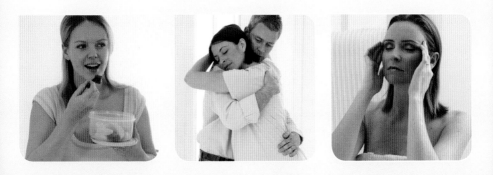

Common complaints

During pregnancy, you may have a number of minor complaints that are irritating but not serious. Most of these are caused by a combination of hormonal changes and the extra strain that your body is experiencing. These can range from aches and pains to changes in your digestion, your sleep patterns, and your mood. They can mostly be treated very simply and are nothing to worry about. A few, however, can be serious,

COMPLAINT	WHY IT HAPPENS
Backache is usually felt as a general discomfort across the lower part of the back, often with pain in the buttocks and down the legs. You can get it when you've been standing in a bad posture for too long, or after lifting something heavy, especially during the third trimester.	High progesterone levels soften and stretch the ligaments of the pelvic bones, thus allowing the baby to be born. The ligaments of the spine also relax, putting extra strain on the joints of the back and hips.
You may also get intensely painful lower backache when you rotate your spine and pelvis in opposite directions, such as when you turn over sideways in bed.	The baby rests against your sacroiliac joint, which is located about 7.5 centimetres (3 inches) in from the top of your buttocks. Rotary movements of the spine and pelvis open and close the sacroiliac joint, and result in pain.
Carpal tunnel syndrome is a sensation of pins and needles, mainly in the thumb and first finger, with numbness and sometimes weakness. Occasionally, the whole hand and forearm is affected. It can occur from conception onwards.	This is caused by pressure on the nerve that passes from the arm to the hand along the front of the wrist. Water retention in the body causes the carpal tunnel (a ring of fibres around the wrist under which the nerve passes) to swell, which in turn exerts pressure on the nerve.
Constipation is when you have dry, hard stools that are difficult to pass. It can occur from conception onwards.	Progesterone relaxes the muscles in the intestinal walls, so there are fewer contractions to push the food along. Consequently, much more water than usual is absorbed from the stool in the colon, making it hard and dry. Stools may also be less frequent.
Cramp is a sudden pain in the thigh, calf, and/or foot, followed by a general ache that lasts for some time. It tends to be more common in the third trimester, and usually wakes you from sleep.	Cramps may be caused by low calcium levels in the blood, or they can occur due to salt deficiency. Check with your doctor.

so be aware of the symptoms and be prepared to act promptly if you suspect all may not be well. Vaginal bleeding at any stage of pregnancy, for example, should always be taken seriously (see p. 70).

If you have a pre-existing medical condition, such as diabetes or AIDS, you will need special monitoring and advice throughout your pregnancy. Make sure your doctor and midwife are aware of your condition. They will give you the advice and support you need.

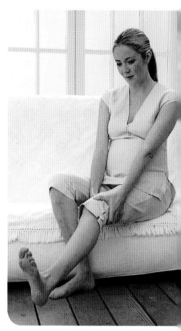

Relieving cramp Keeping your foot flexed, make circling movements with your lower leg, first in one direction, then in the other.

WHAT CAN BE DONE	RISK TO BABY
A massage may help (see p. 40). Do exercises to strengthen your spine. Make sure your mattress is firm. Lift heavy weights correctly. Try to improve your posture and avoid wearing high-heeled shoes. If the pain runs down the back of your leg towards your foot, consult your doctor in case it's a slipped disc. Osteopathic manipulation can help you even in the most severe cases. Backache usually eases by itself in the fifth month when the fetus tips forward – although you may not want to wait that long! If it does not ease, consult a physiotherapist – you may need to wear a supporting belt.	None
You will be given physiotherapy. A splint on the wrist at night may help, as may holding your hand above your head and wiggling your fingers. Acupuncture may help, too. Sleep with your arm on a pillow. Symptoms usually disappear soon after delivery.	None
Drink lots of water. Eat as much roughage in the form of fruit, vegetables, and fibre as you can. Walk briskly for at least 20 minutes a day. Don't take a laxative without consulting your doctor. Natural fibre laxatives are best as they simply increase the amount of water in the stool, making it soft. Figs and prunes will also do the job.	None
Massage the area very firmly. Flex your foot up and push into the heel.	None

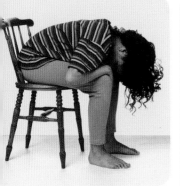

Coping with faintness If you feel faint, put your head as far down as you can – between your knees if you can still manage it! When you feel better, get up slowly.

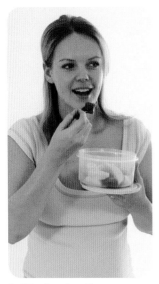

Avoiding heartburn To prevent your stomach from becoming too full, eat smaller meals. Snack on nutritious food and if large meals fill you up, split them into several smaller ones.

Common complaints (continued)

COMPLAINT	WHY IT HAPPENS
Diarrhoea is when you have soft, watery stools, requiring frequent visits to the toilet. It can occur at any time.	It usually occurs because of infection by bacteria or a virus.
Faintness is a feeling of dizziness or vertigo that occurs suddenly, making you unsteady on your feet. It can come on if you stand up too quickly, or have been on your feet for too long, especially in hot weather.	This is due to a lack of blood supply to the brain, often caused by pooling of the blood in the legs and feet when standing, together with the demands of the uterus for an increased blood supply.
Heartburn is a burning sensation just behind the breastbone, sometimes with regurgitation of stomach acid into the mouth. It occurs most commonly while lifting heavy weights, lying down, coughing, or straining when passing a stool.	Early in pregnancy, the muscular valve at the entrance to your stomach relaxes under the influence of progesterone. This allows the stomach acid to flow up into the oesophagus, causing a burning sensation. Later in pregnancy, the baby can press up on the stomach, forcing the contents back into the oesophagus.
High blood pressure (hypertension) is a mild or severe increase in blood pressure. It is usually indicated by symptoms such as headaches, vomiting, and visual disturbances, although some women may experience only a few or none of these. Water retention with swelling of the feet, hands, and ankles may also occur. It can happen at any time, but is more likely to occur near your due date. It is more common in women having their first baby, especially if they are over 35, and also in women having more than one baby. High blood pressure may be a warning of pre-eclampsia (see p. 70).	The cause of hypertension is not fully understood. In some women, cells from the placenta produce chemicals called vasoconstrictors that may cause the blood vessels to constrict. This may lead to a rise in blood pressure and cause the kidneys to retain sodium, in turn leading to water retention.

WHAT CAN BE DONE	RISK TO BABY
Increase your water intake to about 12–14 glasses a day to replace lost fluid. This will ensure that your blood pressure remains normal. Consult your doctor, who will test your stools for infection and give you the appropriate treatment.	Diarrhoea can cause dehydration and loss of calories, which can put your baby at risk if left untreated for a long time. If it is profuse and protracted, you may need to be hospitalized for intravenous feeding.
Avoid standing for long periods. Always sit or lie down when you feel dizzy. Don't get up suddenly after sitting, or get out of a hot bath too quickly. Keep cool in hot weather. If dizzy, sit with your head between your knees – if you still can – or lie down with your feet higher than your head.	None, unless you fall very heavily on to your stomach.
Eat small meals so that your stomach is never too full. Sleep propped up with several pillows. A glass of milk at bedtime will help neutralize stomach acid. Your doctor may also prescribe antacids, and these can be safely taken throughout your pregnancy.	None
If you suffered from high blood pressure before you were pregnant, tell your doctor. Keep an eye on your weight. Make sure that you report any persistent headaches and nausea. Your doctor will test your blood pressure and urine, and look for any swelling (see p. 68) of your hands, face, and ankles at each antenatal visit. If your blood pressure goes up at any stage of the pregnancy, you'll almost certainly have to see your doctor more often and you may be asked to attend the antenatal day unit at the hospital for checking. If the rise is severe, you'll need to go into the hospital, where you can be monitored continuously. If your baby appears to be suffering, your labour may be induced or you may have a Caesarean section. The blood pressure usually returns to normal once your baby is born.	Pregnancy-induced hypertension or pre-eclampsia (see p. 70) can slow the baby's growth rate, as blood flow to the uterus gets reduced. Your baby could also be short of oxygen. Both these factors may lead to low birthweight. The severe form of this, called eclampsia, can be life-threatening. Fortunately, this is now rare in the West because of the excellent antenatal care available, with symptoms being spotted at an early stage.

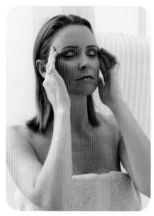

Self-massage Massaging your face, temples, and neck is an effective way of relieving tension and may help dispel insomnia.

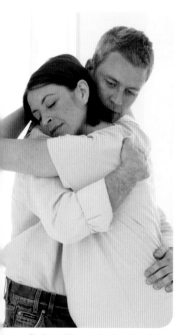

Coping with mood swings A quick, reassuring cuddle is probably just what you need when you're feeling anxious and upset.

Common complaints (continued)

COMPLAINT	WHY IT HAPPENS
Insomnia is the inability to sleep at night, which makes you tired and irritable during the day. It can happen at any time from conception onwards.	Your baby lives on a 24-hour clock, with a metabolism that keeps going even when you want to sleep. This can affect your body's responses. Other causes include night sweats, difficulty in getting comfortable, and a need to empty your bladder more frequently, particularly during the third trimester.
Mood swings are uncharacteristic, rapid changes in mood, often with unexplained crying and anxiety attacks. They are common from conception onwards, but are especially likely to occur in the third trimester.	Changes in your hormonal balance during pregnancy have a depressant effect on the nervous system, causing symptoms similar to those that you may experience before your period. A change to your self-image and a possible identity crisis may also have a profound effect on you when you're pregnant. Mixed feelings about pregnancy and parenthood can also cause sudden shifts in your moods.
Morning sickness is a feeling of nausea, sometimes accompanied by vomiting. Contrary to its name, it can occur at any time of the day, but is most common when you haven't eaten for a long time, or after a full night's sleep. It generally occurs in the first trimester, and eases off later on.	The main cause is low blood sugar, but pregnancy hormones may irritate the stomach directly.
Piles are dilated veins in the rectum (for varicose veins – see p. 68) that may protrude from the anus. They usually do not develop until the second trimester of pregnancy.	Your growing baby presses down on your rectum and impedes blood flow to the heart. The blood therefore pools, causing the veins to dilate to accommodate the dammed-up blood.

WHAT CAN BE DONE	RISK TO BABY
A warm bath and a hot milky drink may help, as may a relaxing massage (see p. 40). Watch television or read until you feel tired and sleepy. Find a comfortable position, and try to stay cool. Doctors very rarely prescribe sleeping pills in pregnancy because they can cross the placenta and affect the baby.	None
As long as depression doesn't become the dominant mood, you should consider these feelings as natural. Temporary depression, anxiety, and confusion can occur even in the easiest of pregnancies. Talk to your partner about your worries and if you cannot cope, talk to your doctor. (See also p. 42.)	None
Food can provide relief from nausea, so eat little and often. Eat high carbohydrate foods, such as bread, pasta, potatoes, rice, and cereals, which provide long-lasting energy, and avoid fatty foods and coffee. Keep away from cigarette smoke and other strong smells as these can also trigger nausea. Glucose sweets can help, so keep some in your car, desk, or handbag. To prevent morning sickness, put a glass of water and a plain biscuit or two by your bed before sleeping, and have them 15 minutes before you get up in the morning. Drink extra fluids, such as fruit juice or skimmed milk – if you can keep them down.	In its severe form (called *hyperemesis gravidarum*), excessive vomiting can deplete your body's fluid and mineral levels, leading to low blood pressure. This is always harmful to your baby. Inform your doctor if you vomit more than three times a day for three days. In very severe cases, hospitalization may be necessary to replace the fluids that you have lost.
Keep your bowels regular and the stools soft by eating sufficient fibre – this will help you avoid straining. Don't lift weights, as this will increase pressure on your abdomen and in the rectal veins. Have coughs treated promptly for the same reasons. Aromatherapy may help relieve some symptoms.	None

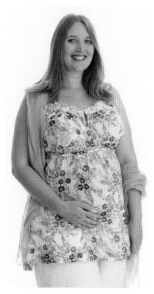

Comfortable clothing You should wear loose-fitting, comfortable clothes when you are pregnant, as tight-fitting clothing will constrict you.

Common complaints (continued)

COMPLAINT	WHY IT HAPPENS
Rib pain can be felt as extreme soreness and tenderness of the ribs, usually on the right side, just below the breasts. The pain is more severe when you sit down. It tends to occur mainly during the third trimester.	It is caused by pressure on the ribs as the baby grows in the abdomen. In addition, the baby can bruise your lower ribs with his head, or by excessive punching and kicking.
Tender, painful breasts that feel heavy and uncomfortable, with a tingling in the nipples, can be one of the first signs of pregnancy. Your breasts may be tender and painful throughout, but these signs usually worsen towards term.	Hormones are preparing your breasts for lactation. The milk ducts are growing and being stretched as they fill with milk.
Thrush is a thick, white, curdy discharge from the vagina, accompanied by dryness and intense itching around your vulva, perineum, vagina, and sometimes, your anus. You may also feel pain while passing urine.	Thrush is an infection caused by the yeast *Candida albicans*, which occurs normally in the bowel. Infection occurs when the yeast grows uncontrolled by other bacteria, perhaps after a course of antibiotics. Though thrush can happen at any time, it is most common in pregnancy. Excess sugar intake often aggravates it.
Varicose veins are swollen veins just below the skin. Although most common in the legs or anus, they can also develop in the vulva.	These are caused by the same mechanism as piles (see p. 66).
Water retention happens when there is an increase in the amount of fluid present in the tissues. This causes swelling (oedema), especially of the ankles, feet, face, and hands. Remove your rings before they become too tight.	Standing all day, especially in hot weather, can cause fluid to pool in the ankles and feet. High blood pressure (see p. 64), which is a common problem in pregnancy, can force fluid from the bloodstream into the tissues, causing swelling and puffiness. Pregnancy hormones can cause the kidneys to retain sodium, in turn leading to water retention by the body.

WHAT CAN BE DONE	RISK TO BABY
Wear loose clothes that don't restrict your ribs. Improve your posture – try not to slump forwards when sitting. Prop yourself up on cushions when you lie down. The pain eases when the baby's head drops into the pelvic cavity prior to labour.	None
Wear a good supportive bra from early in pregnancy. If your breasts become very large, wear a bra at night as well (see p. 53). To prevent soreness, wash your breasts gently once a day with a mild soap and pat dry. Apply baby lotion or oil to your nipples if they become sore and dry.	None
Avoid wearing tight underwear and trousers, as this encourages infection. Choose cotton underwear instead of items made from synthetic fibres. The doctor will prescribe pessaries that you should place in your vagina at night, as directed. You will also be prescribed a cream that should be gently rubbed into the skin around your vaginal opening and anus. These treatments should stop the discharge and thus the itching.	None
Don't stand for long periods. Put your feet up whenever you can. Wear pregnancy support tights. Gentle massage of the legs may help prevent varicose veins, but do not massage the area if you have already developed them.	None
Avoid standing for prolonged periods. Whenever possible, put your feet up. Try not to eat salty foods too much. Your doctor will check your hands, face, and ankles for any swelling at each antenatal visit. Diuretics are not recommended during pregnancy.	In extreme forms, this can be potentially dangerous (see pre-eclampsia, p. 70).

When to get concerned

Vaginal bleeding at any stage of pregnancy should be taken seriously. It may indicate an abnormally placed placenta, placenta praevia (see right), or a warning that a miscarriage is imminent. Both conditions require prompt treatment.

However, vaginal bleeding occurs in the first trimester in about a quarter of all pregnancies. Over half of these continue, and end with the delivery of a healthy baby.

If you start to bleed during the second or third trimester, call your maternity unit and go there as soon as you can.

Pre-eclampsia Unique to pregnancy, this illness may occur in as many as 1 in 10 pregnancies and affects both mother and baby. It occurs most often in a first pregnancy or in a multiple pregnancy, usually in the second half of pregnancy. The exact cause is unknown, although the risk is greatest if there is a family history.

It is potentially dangerous for the baby because the placenta becomes deficient and raises the mother's blood pressure, both of which can happen silently – often the first sign is swelling of the ankles, face, and fingers. Another sign is protein in the urine. Untreated, the condition can progress to coma and fits, and be a threat to the baby's life. Delivery is the only solution.

Medical conditions

The vast majority of pregnancies proceed to term without problems or emergencies. However, there are certain medical conditions that require careful monitoring and treatment during pregnancy.

Placenta praevia This is the medical term for the condition when the placenta is positioned "ahead of" the baby in the uterus. During labour it could prevent the baby's head from descending, or even if the placenta is not blocking the way it could become dislodged and bleed.

If placenta praevia is suspected, you'll have an ultrasound scan early on and if confirmed, at term or even slightly earlier (38 weeks), your baby will be delivered by Caesarean section.

Diabetes Diabetic mothers deliver normal, healthy babies most of the time – so as long as the diabetes is well controlled throughout your pregnancy, it poses little threat to you or your baby. If you're an established diabetic, you'll be monitored closely throughout pregnancy and your dose of insulin will need to be adjusted.

Pregnancy can "unmask" a tendency to develop gestational diabetes, which can be controlled through diet, and which normally disappears after delivery. Babies of diabetic mothers can grow very large and if yours does, you may be induced before term so that he can still be born vaginally. At antenatal visits, your blood sugar, blood pressure, and urine are checked, and your diet carefully monitored.

HIV Being HIV positive shouldn't affect your pregnancy, nor will pregnancy necessarily precipitate AIDS in yourself. Pregnancy, however, does alter your immune state and you're less able to fight infections.

You must take care of yourself in terms of eating well, staying fit, and getting enough rest. Nowadays, you'll be given special care and will probably have several specialists as well as your midwife caring for you. Your condition can remain confidential.

Your baby is at a risk of being infected with the virus, but taking anti-viral drugs ensures that the amount of virus in your system is very low and the risks to the baby are minimal.

Chapter 6

Your sensual pregnancy

The physical, mental, and emotional
changes you undergo during pregnancy
can influence your attitude to sex, but
there is no need to allow pregnancy to
displace sensuality in your relationship.

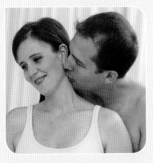
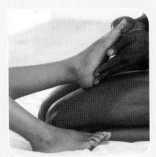
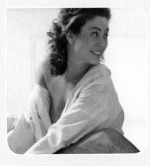

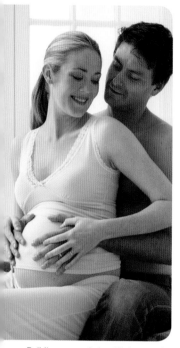

Building your relationship Love and understanding will help to minimize any problems that may arise due to the physical and emotional changes that take place during pregnancy.

Your new sensuality

It's perfectly safe to enjoy sex during your pregnancy, unless there are medical reasons why you should abstain. Moreover, every pregnant woman has the potential to enjoy sex possibly more than she ever has before.

The desire for sex and the enjoyment of it varies widely, not only from one woman to another during pregnancy, but also in the same woman at different times throughout its duration. Typically, though, there is a decline in interest in sex during the first trimester (especially if you are suffering from tiredness and nausea), followed by an increase in the second trimester, with another decline in the third trimester.

When a pregnant woman does have sex, she may find it far more exciting and satisfying than it was before she conceived. In fact, a woman will sometimes achieve orgasm or multiple orgasms for the first time when she is pregnant. This enhanced sexuality is principally because of the high levels of female hormones and pregnancy hormones that circulate throughout her body when she is pregnant (see p. 73). These cause a number of important changes to her breasts and sexual organs, making them more sensitive and responsive.

Eroticism during pregnancy

One of the effects of the rise in oestrogen levels during pregnancy is an increase in blood flow, especially in the pelvic area. Because of this, the vagina and its folds (the labia) become slightly stretched and swollen. This stretching and swelling, which normally occurs only during sexual excitement, makes the sensory nerve endings hypersensitive, resulting in rapid arousal.

The breasts start to enlarge almost as soon as pregnancy occurs and one of the classic signs of pregnancy is sensitive, enlarged breasts with nipples that may tingle or even feel painful. The increased sensitivity of the breasts makes them a focus of sensory arousal, and a woman can feel enhanced sensations when her nipples and breasts are caressed and kissed by her partner. This sexual foreplay can also result in the arousal of the clitoris and the vagina.

Because of the increased blood flow, the vaginal secretions are quite profuse, so a pregnant woman usually becomes ready for penetration much earlier than usual. Penetration is particularly easy because of this, and a climax can be achieved quite quickly if the clitoris is stimulated simultaneously. The intensity of orgasm may reach new heights and the time taken to "come down" from an orgasm can be greatly extended. This is evident in the labia minora and the lower end of the vagina, which can remain swollen for anything up to two hours after orgasm, particularly in the last trimester.

Incidental to stimulating the whole of the genital area, the pregnancy hormones stimulate the production of a hormone that results in deeper skin pigmentation – particularly in the nipple area. Darkening of the nipples can act as a sexual signal to a man, making his partner's breasts very attractive to him.

When to make love

You can make love whenever you want to, as long as it's not too athletic and there are no medical reasons for you to forego it. Good sex in pregnancy helps prepare you for childbirth by keeping your pelvic muscles strong and supple. As at any other time, it also bonds you closer to your partner, which will help you cope much better with the stresses of parenthood.

There is absolutely no physical reason why a woman having a normal pregnancy should not enjoy sexual relations with her partner to the full and, if both partners are willing, sex need not stop any earlier than the onset of labour. In a low-risk pregnancy, the uterine spasms that accompany orgasms are perfectly safe, and in late pregnancy may be beneficial because they help prepare the uterus for the rigours of labour.

It is a fallacy that sex can cause an infection during pregnancy and may harm the baby – infection is virtually impossible because the cervix is closed and has a tough mucus plug that prevents the ascent of bacteria into the uterus. In addition, the baby is completely enclosed within the amniotic sac, which resists rupture even when under great pressure and cushions the baby against all external forces (including the weight of your partner during intercourse).

Extremely athletic sex is not a good idea, because it may cause soreness and abrasions and a pregnant woman should be free of these unnecessary discomforts. Try to understand any changes in your own and your partner's sexual desires, and be open with each other when discussing your needs. But never allow your sex life to become the dominant feature of your relationship. Concentrate on loving rather than lovemaking, and if at any time you or your partner don't feel like sex, rediscover the intimacy and joy of simply being with the one you love.

Your hormonal changes

A woman undergoes many physical, psychological, and emotional changes during pregnancy, which will influence her attitude to sex and her enjoyment of it. These changes are due mainly to the vastly increased levels of hormones circulating in her body.

The most important hormones involved in maintaining pregnancy are progesterone and oestrogen. In the early days of a pregnancy these are produced by the *corpus luteum* in the ovary. However, once the embryo has implanted in the womb lining, the developing placenta takes over as the primary source of progesterone and oestrogen.

The increase in the amounts of these hormones circulating in the body is swift and dramatic. The level of progesterone rises to 10 times what it was before conception, while the amount of oestrogen produced in a single day is equivalent to that generated by a non-pregnant woman's ovaries in three years. In fact, during the course of a single pregnancy, a woman will produce as much oestrogen as a non-pregnant woman could in 150 years.

Progesterone and oestrogen induce a sense of wellbeing. They also lead to shining hair, and supple and glowing skin. They create an aura of tranquillity and contentment.

Your partner's do's and don'ts

By making a few adjustments to your lovemaking, you can make the experience happier for the mother-to-be.

Do:

✳ Be tender, romantic, patient, and understanding.

✳ Use different kinds of stroking, such as a firm hand over her abdomen if the baby is kicking.

✳ Keep your weight off her stomach and breasts when making love.

✳ Use lots of pillows for greater comfort and to get the right angles around the curves of her body.

✳ Take your time while you are making love, and don't be afraid to experiment.

Don't:

✳ Force her to make love if she doesn't feel like it.

✳ Expect her to have simultaneous orgasms – or even one orgasm.

Making love

You can continue making love as late into pregnancy as you wish, as long as there are no medical reasons for refraining from it (see p. 76). Your baby, safe within your uterus, cannot be harmed by any normal sexual activity, and probably enjoys sex as much as you do because your hormones reach him through the placenta.

In the early months you can use any lovemaking position you choose, but as your abdomen swells you will probably find that making love in some positions, particularly the missionary position, with your partner on top, becomes uncomfortable. You may have to change your sexual habits, and the best way to approach this change is to realize that it is an opportunity to build on and enhance the physical side of your relationship.

As your pregnancy advances, there are plenty of other erotic and exciting positions you can try. For instance, both of you can explore (perhaps for the first time) the pleasures of new lovemaking positions and of other forms of sexual activity, such as mutual masturbation and oral sex. These alternatives are also often the best options when you first resume lovemaking after the birth of your baby.

Woman-on-top positions

You will probably find these positions most comfortable from the second trimester onwards. As your abdomen enlarges, you can lift yourself further off your partner's stomach by supporting yourself on your knees. In this way, you can avoid too much pressure on the abdomen and breasts. Also, in these positions, you can better control the depth of your partner's penetration as well as the speed and rhythm of your lovemaking.

These positions allow a great deal of intimacy. You and your partner have your hands free to caress and stroke each other and he can easily reach your breasts with his mouth. Alternatively, you can brush his chest with your breasts to stimulate him further.

Kneeling and side-by-side positions

These positions, many of which involve entering from behind, can be adopted especially during pregnancy. They are particularly useful if you don't feel very comfortable lying flat on your back, or at those times when you do not want to take too active a part in the lovemaking.

Kneeling positions allow your partner much freedom of movement and let him vary the amount of penetration. Side-by-side positions are not only comfortable and pleasurable, but permit plenty of passionate kissing and caressing. The "spoons" position, which is so called because the partners nestle together like a pair of spoons, will also be useful if you experience any soreness or discomfort when you resume lovemaking after you have given birth, especially if you have had a tear or an episiotomy during labour.

A variation on this position, with the woman lying on her back on top of her partner, frees her from any pressure on her abdomen while her partner has complete access to her vagina. He can continue to stimulate her either with his hand or his penis.

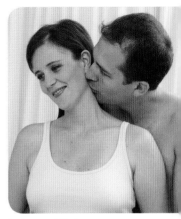

Loving touch During pregnancy, when sex is not as easy or desirable as before, touching, kissing, and cuddling are ways of maintaining the loving bonds between a couple.

Sitting positions

Most useful in the middle and late months, these positions don't allow a lot of movement but they are comfortable for both partners and lessen pressure on the abdomen. In addition, the depth of penetration can be controlled. In these positions, your partner sits on a sturdy, comfortable chair or on the edge of the bed and you sit on his lap, either facing him (if your abdomen is not too big), facing to one side, or facing away from him.

When you are facing to one side or away from your partner, he can use his hands to caress your body and breasts and to stimulate your clitoris. In addition, because his range of movement is limited, you have control of the sexual tempo.

Anxieties

Even without a pregnancy and the attendant emotional and physical adjustments you both need to make, everyone experiences difficulties in their love life from time to time. There are reasons enough for any woman to feel weary in pregnancy – a disappearing waistline, sore breasts, abdominal discomfort, the need to empty the bladder frequently all militate against passionate sex. In addition, the man (and sometimes both partners) may fear that sex can somehow harm the baby (it can't – if anything your baby enjoys it). Talking things over, however, is essential, not only to explore different options and find comfortable positions but also to discuss your feelings about the move from partnership into parenthood.

When sex may be inadvisable

If yours is a high-risk pregnancy, you may need to avoid sex at certain times, or even completely.

Your doctor will warn you if there is any risk of sexual activity being a danger to your pregnancy, and advise you on what is safe – and when. You should always make sure that he or she explains the problem fully, so that you are completely clear about what you can and cannot safely do.

The most common reasons and times for restricting sexual intercourse during pregnancy include the following:

✳ Whenever there is any sign of bleeding: the bleeding may well be quite harmless, but you should consult your doctor without delay.

✳ If you have a history of miscarriage in the first trimester, or if you are showing signs that you might miscarry early in pregnancy.

✳ If placenta praevia (see p. 70) is suspected or confirmed.

✳ In the last trimester of a multiple pregnancy.

✳ In the last 12 weeks, if you have a history of premature labour, or if you are showing signs that you might go into premature labour.

✳ If your waters have broken.

Sexual problems

When you are pregnant, a number of physical and emotional factors may lessen the pleasure of having sex. Fortunately, only a few of these actually prevent you from having intercourse, and they are relatively rare (see column, left).

Lowered sex drive

Many women feel that their bodies become less and less attractive as pregnancy progresses, and this lack of confidence about their appearance often leads to a lowered inclination for sex. It is also difficult to feel attractive and sexy if you're suffering from the nausea and extreme fatigue of early pregnancy. In the second trimester, once free of these distractions, most women find that their interest and pleasure in sex returns. Towards the end of pregnancy, though, libido may wane again, largely due once more to fatigue.

Hormone levels can swing quite violently during pregnancy, and you may find that you're emotionally volatile, switching from contentment to sadness and tearfulness, and then to great elation. All this is perfectly normal but, of course, it can have an adverse effect on your sexual relationship with your partner. If it does, you must be open with him and honest about your feelings – and if you don't want to make love because you feel physically ill or excessively tired, tell him why, otherwise he could easily feel responsible, or worse, that you're rejecting him.

Discomfort

As pregnancy progresses, partly as a result of high oestrogen levels and partly due to fluid retention, your body becomes very sensitive to touch, especially the breasts, labia, and outer part of the vagina. This can mean that you have a heightened sexual response (see p. 72), but sometimes, this sensitivity can verge on tenderness, and foreplay may be unpleasant. Explain this to your partner and ask him to avoid touching these tender areas. Your engorged genitals may become swollen and aching after orgasm, and can remain so for some time. This can cause a feeling of unrelieved fullness, which may make sex less satisfying. The sexual positions you used to enjoy earlier may become extremely uncomfortable now. A little experimentation with non-penetrative sex, mutual masturbation, and new positions may be the answer.

Useful addresses

Advice on general health

British Acupuncture Council
63 Jeddo Road
London W12 9HQ
Tel: 020 8735 0400
www.acupuncture.org.uk

British Epilepsy Association
New Anstey House
Gate Way Drive
Yeadon, Leeds LS19 7XY
Tel: 0113 210 8800
www.epilepsy.org.uk

British Homeopathic Association
Hahnemann House
29 Park Street West
Luton LU1 3BE
Tel: 01582 408675
www.britishhhomeopathic.org

Diabetes UK (formerly the British
Diabetic Association)
Macleod House
10 Parkway
London NW1 7AA
Tel: 020 7424 1000
www.diabetes.org.uk

The National Asthma Campaign
Summit House
70 Wilson Street
London EC2A 2DB
Tel: 0800 121 62 44
www.asthma.org.uk

The National Eczema Society
Hill House
Highgate Hill
London N19 5NA
Tel: 0870 241 3604
www.eczema.org

Advice on pregnancy and childbirth

Caesarean Support Network
55 Cooil Drive
Douglas
Isle of Man IM2 2HF
Tel: 01624 661269 (after 6 pm)

National Childbirth Trust
Alexandra House
Oldham Terrace, Acton
London W3 6NH
Tel: 0870 770 3236
www.netpregnancyandbabycare.com

APEC (Action on Pre-eclampsia)
2c The Halfcraft, Syston LE7 1LD
Tel: 020 8427 4217
www.apec.org.uk

Birthworks
14–15 Fiddlebridge Industrial Centre
Hatfield, Hertfordshire AL10 0DE
Tel: 01707 880333
www.birthworks.org

Advice and literature on water births, birth pools for hire

Aqua Birth Pools, Active Birth Centre
Bickerton House, 25 Bickerton Road
London N19 5JT
Tel: 020 7281 6760
www.activebirthcentre.com

Advice and consultation on infertility and miscarriage

St Mary's Hospital Recurrent
Miscarriage Clinic
Winston Churchill Wing
Praed Street London W2 1NY
Tel: 020 7886 7777

Advice on the care of children with Down's syndrome

Down's Syndrome Association
Langdon Down Centre
2a Langdon Park
Teddington TW11 9PS
Tel: 020 8682 4001
www.downs-syndrome.org.uk

Nationwide antenatal classes and practical postnatal help

RCOG (Royal College of Obstetricians
and Gynaecologists)
27 Sussex Place, Regent's Park
London NW1 4RG
Tel: 020 7772 6200
www.rcog.org.uk

Royal College of Midwives
15 Mansfield Street
London W1G 9NH
Tel: 020 7312 3535
www.rcm.org.uk

Advice on reproductive health

Women's Health
52 Featherstone Street
London EC1Y 8RT
Tel: 020 7251 6580

National support network for bereaved parents

SANDS (Stillbirth and Neonatal
Death Society)
28 Portland Place
London W1B 1LY
Tel: 020 7436 5881

Support for multiple births

TAMBA (Twins and Multiple
Birth Association)
2 The Willows
Gardner Road
Guildford
Surrey GU1 4PG
Tel: 0870 770 3305
www.tamba.org.uk

Nutritional advice for pregnant women who are vegetarians

Vegetarian Society
Parkdale Dunham Road
Altrincham
Cheshire WA14 4QG
Tel: 0161 925 2000
www.vegsoc.org

Pressure group for parents to have the maternity services they want

AIMS (Association for Improvements
in Maternity Services)
5 Ann's Court
Grove Road
Surbiton
Surrey KT6 4BE
Tel: 0208 390 9534
www.aims.org.uk

24-hour telephone service for mothers (Supplies network of breastfeeding counsellors)

Association of Breastfeeding Mothers
PO Box 207
Bridgwater,
Somerset TA6 7YT
Tel: 0870 401 7711
www.abm.me.uk

Index

Acknowledgments

DK would like to thank Dr Elizabeth Owen, for consulting on medical issues, and Angela Baynham, for proofreading.

The publisher would like to thank the following for their kind permission to reproduce their photographs:

Getty Images: Sri Maiava Rusden page 8; Ian Hooton page 10; **Mother & Baby Picture Library**: Ian Hooton page 20; **Science Photo Library**: Hattie Young page 12

All other images © Dorling Kindersley For further information see: www.dkimages.com.